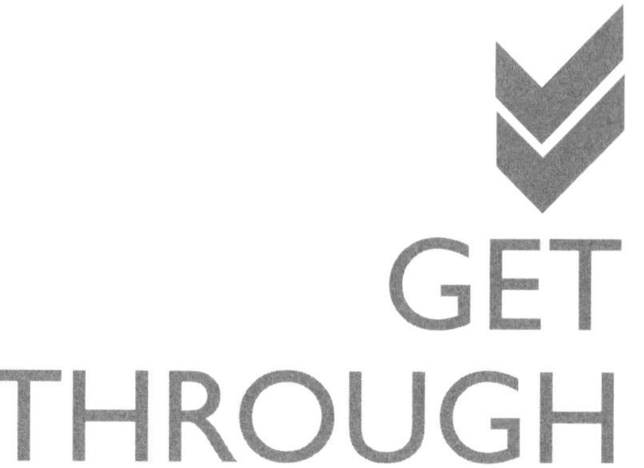

GET THROUGH

Primary FRCA: SBAs

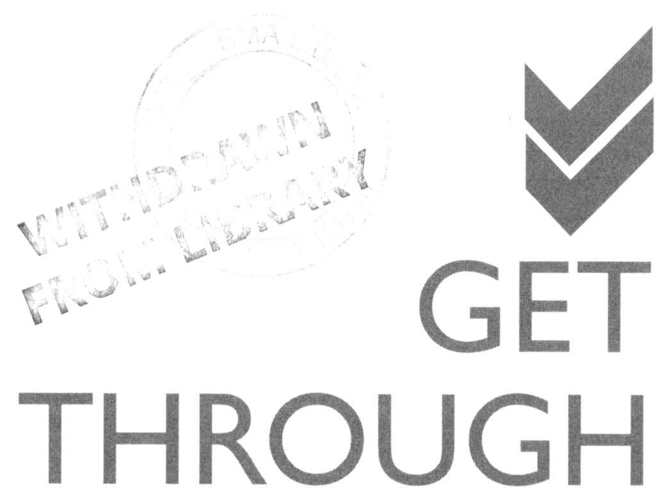

Primary FRCA: SBAs

Desikan Rangarajan FRCA PhD
Speciality Registrar in Anaesthesia, The Royal London Hospital
Barts Health NHS Trust, London, UK

Mandeep Phull FRCA BSc
Speciality Registrar in Anaesthesia, The Royal London Hospital
Barts Health NHS Trust, London, UK

Vinodkumar Patil FRCA
Honorary Senior Clinical Lecturer,
Queen Mary, University of London, London, UK,
and Consultant in Anaesthesia,
BHR University Hospitals NHS Trust
Romford, UK

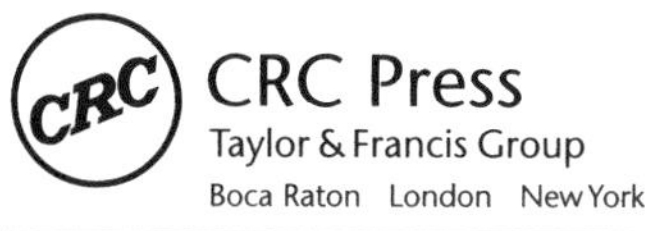
CRC Press
Taylor & Francis Group
Boca Raton London New York

CRC Press is an imprint of the
Taylor & Francis Group, an **informa** business

CRC Press
Taylor & Francis Group
6000 Broken Sound Parkway NW, Suite 300
Boca Raton, FL 33487-2742

Printed on acid-free paper
Version Date: 20130716

International Standard Book Number-13: 978-1-4441-7606-3 (Paperback)

Library of Congress Cataloging-in-Publication Data

Rangarajan, Desikan (Anesthesiologist), author.
Get through primary FRCA : SBAs / Desikan Rangarajan, Mandeep Phull, Vinodkumar Patil.
p. ; cm. -- (Get through)
Includes bibliographical references and index.
ISBN 978-1-4441-7606-3 (paperback : alk. paper)
I. Phull, Mandeep, author. II. Patil, Vinodkumar, author. III. Title. IV. Series: Get through.
[DNLM: 1. Anesthesia--Examination Questions. WO 218.2]

RD82.3
617.9'6076--dc23 2013019698

Visit the Taylor & Francis Web site at
http://www.taylorandfrancis.com

and the CRC Press Web site at
http://www.crcpress.com

CONTENTS

FOREWORD

Anaesthetists have always been at the leading edge of ensuring the delivery of safe, high quality clinical practices. It is recognised that quality training translates to a high quality practitioner. The Royal College of Anaesthetists (RCoA) has been at the heart of maintaining standards and producing high quality anaesthetists by developing curricula that are 'fit for purpose', and assessment processes that are relevant. Postgraduate exams remain a key component in the assessment of competence in all specialties and continue to be important in maintaining standards of clinical care. The Fellowship of the Royal College of Anaesthetist is still prized by anaesthetists in training in both the UK and around the world. It is recognized as a mark of high quality training and a significant professional achievement.

The FRCA exam continues to be reviewed and adapted; an example of this being the introduction of the single best answer component to the Primary exam in 2011. This was introduced in response to criticisms from the Postgraduate Medical Education and Training Board (PMETB) that the traditional multiple choice question exam tested factual recall only but not the ability to apply that knowledge. The single best answer (SBA) had been adopted by a number of other postgraduate medical exams, and the RCoA subsequently agreed to introduce this method of assessment into the FRCA exam. This represented a major undertaking of work for examiners and others in writing new questions, something I was privileged to be part of as an examiner at that time.

The SBA is considered a better assessment of 'knows how' *and* 'knows why' rather than just 'knows' and could be more discriminatory in reducing the impact of guesswork. At time of writing, the RCoA has published the results of three sittings of the Primary exam containing SBA. Analysis of these sittings demonstrated that combining the SBA with traditional multiple choice questions did not reduce the pass rate, and if anything may have increased it marginally.

Due to the relative recent introduction of SBA questions, there are few practice texts for the Primary exam. This book is therefore timely and I am sure will prove useful to candidates revising for the exam. The authors have devised a wide range of questions, (both single best answers and single correct answers) with a range of subject matter from basic science to clinical practice. The answers come with useful explanations and with references which help the reader delve into the subject in further depth should they wish to do so.

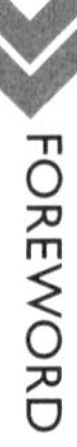

I wish all of you aspiring anaesthetists and perioperative care physicians success in your forthcoming exam and your future career. You have chosen an excellent career to follow.

Dr Arun K Gupta, MBBS, MA, PhD, FFICM, FRCA, FHEA
Director of Postgraduate Education
Academic Health Sciences Centre
Cambridge University Health Partners
Director of Postgraduate Medical Education
Director of the Addenbrooke's Simulation Centre
Consultant in Anaesthesia and Neurointensive Care
Cambridge University Hospitals
Associate Lecturer, University of Cambridge

PREFACE

A broad knowledge base is a prerequisite to function as a competent anaesthetist, and the FRCA primary syllabus reflects this requirement. Indeed, the extensive breadth and depth of knowledge expected are daunting and at times may appear insurmountable. Furthermore, there has been a trend in recent years to sit and pass the examination as early as possible, so as to facilitate successful competition for training numbers. Such a trend limits candidates' ability to add to their knowledge by experience, and more and more emphasis is placed on book work.

It cannot be overemphasised that preparation is key to passing this exam. We would advocate that the candidate plan well ahead and read voraciously. Though detailed knowledge is desirable, a broad understanding on extensive topics is likely to help the candidate in the first instance. We feel that layering of information is without doubt the best approach; the basic foundation of concepts should be sound before the addition of details. For example, it is better to know how the oil–gas partition value of a particular anaesthetic agent relates to potency, rather than to know the actual value without appreciation of the significance. Once the foundations are solid, candidates will find it easy to pin additional information, which thus allows them to tackle seemingly impossible questions and also to impress examiners in the oral component of the exam. Bear in mind that this process takes time, and do not be discouraged in the early part of your endeavour. You are not alone.

A shrewd mid-sixteenth-century European proverb states, 'Use makes perfect,' and as such practice papers should be incorporated into the preparation for the written component of the Primary FRCA examination. Practice papers allow candidates to not only test their knowledge but also become familiar with the format and time limits. The Single Best Answer (SBA) has only recently been introduced into the Primary FRCA examinations. The SBAs comprise one third of the marks available in the written paper, and hence there is scope to lose a substantial number of points should the candidate be ill prepared. Our personal observations indicate that candidates struggle with the SBA format, and many have failed the written component of the Primary FRCA examination as a consequence. To compound this, there are few sources in print that aid candidates to appreciate the complexity of such questions.

We have set about to address this issue by compiling an examination aid which contains six papers, each containing 30 SBA questions. The chief aim of this book is to expose the candidate to the format and provide a safe environment in which to practice and prepare. We have scoured the Primary syllabus to identify topics and have tried to cover all the main headings (Pharmacology, Physiology, Physics, Equipment, Measurement and Clinical scenarios) that are likely to appear as SBAs.

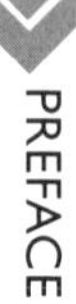

In addition, we have given detailed explanations which not only justify the correct answer but also provide key knowledge on the subject tested. We hope this will add to candidates' understanding. We also expect that this examination aid will enable candidates to spotlight deficits in their knowledge and so aid in targeted last-minute preparation.

All the authors are Fellows of the Royal College of Anaesthetists, and two of the authors have had first-hand experience in answering the SBAs in the FRCA Final examination. We have researched, written, discussed and rewritten the Primary topics and questions in this book. This reflects many months of our free time, and the process has been cathartic. We have reacquainted ourselves with the basic science principles which underpin much of our clinical practice. We hope that you will gain at least as much, if not more, from our endeavour.

We wish you much success.

Dr Desikan Rangarajan, FRCA
Dr Mandeep Phull, FRCA
Dr Vinod Patil, FRCA

ABBREVIATIONS

2,3-DPG	2,3-diphosphoglycerate
A&E	accident and emergency (department of a hospital)
ABG	arterial blood gas
AC	alternating current
ACE	angiotensin-converting enzyme
ACH	acetylcholine
ACTH	adenocorticotrophic hormone
AH	absolute humidity
AIDS	acquired immunodeficiency syndrome
APL	adjustable pressure-limiting
APLS	advanced paediatric life support
APTT	activated partial thromboplastin time
ASA	American Society of Anesthesiologists
AV	atrioventricular
AVRT	atrioventricular re-entrant tachycardia
AZT	azidothymidine
BE	base excess
BiPAP	bi-level positive airway pressure
BMI	body mass index
BMR	basal metabolic rate
BP	blood pressure
cAMP	cyclic adenosine monophosphate
CJD	Creutzfeldt–Jakob disease
CMV	cytomegalovirus
CN	cranial nerve
CNS	central nervous system
COMT	catechol-O-methyltransferase
COPD	chronic obstructive pulmonary disease
CPAP	continuous positive airway pressure
CPR	cardiopulmonary resuscitation
CSF	cerebrospinal fluid
CT	computed tomography
CVP	central venous pressure
CVS	cardiovascular system
CXR	chest X-ray
DBS	double burst stimulation
DC	direct current

DIC	disseminated intravascular coagulopathy
DNA	deoxyribonucleic acid
DRC	dose–response curve
DV	ductus venosus
ECF	extracellular fluid
ECG	electrocardiogram
ECHO	echocardiography
EEG	electroencephalogram
etCO_2	end tidal carbon dioxide
ETT	endotracheal tube
EVD	external ventricular drain
FBC	full blood count
FDA	Food and Drug Administration
FE	fat embolism
FFP	fresh frozen plasma
FGF	fresh gas flow
FRC	functional residual capacity
FRCA	Examination of the Diploma of Fellowship of the British Royal College of Anaesthetists
GABA	gamma amino butyric acid
GCS	Glasgow coma score
GDP	guanine diphosphate
GFR	glomerular filtration rate
GTN	glyceryl trinitrate
GTP	guanine triphosphate
Hb	haemoglobin
HDU	high-dependency unit
HIV	human immunodeficiency virus
HPA	hypothalamic–pituitary axis
ICF	intracellular fluid
ICP	intracranial pressure
ICU	intensive care unit
IDDM	insulin-dependent diabetes mellitus
IgG	immunoglobulin G
IM	intramuscular
ITU	intensive therapy unit
IV	intravenous
LDL	low-density lipoprotein
LMA	laryngeal mask airway
LMWH	low-molecular-weight heparin
LSCS	lower section Caesarean section
MAC	minimum alveolar concentration
MAC	monitored anaesthesia care
MAO	monoamine oxidase
MCV	mean corpuscular volume
MH	malignant hyperthermia
MHRA	Medicines and Healthcare Products Regulatory Agency

mmHg	millimetres of mercury
MRI	magnetic resonance imaging
mRNA	messenger RNA
NICE	National Institute for Health and Care Excellence
NG	nasogastric
NIDDM	non-insulin dependent diabetes mellitus
NM	neuromuscular
NNT	number needed to treat
NO	nitric oxide
NSAID	non-steroidal anti-inflammatory drug
OMV	Oxford miniature vaporizer
ORIF	open reduction and internal fixation
$PaCO_2$	arterial carbon dioxide tension
PaO_2	arterial blood gas
PCA	patient-controlled analgesia
pCO_2	carbon dioxide partial pressure
PDPH	post-dural puncture headache
PEEP	positive end-expiratory pressure
pO_2	oxygen partial pressure
Primary FRCA	Primary Examination of the Diploma of Fellowship of the British Royal College of Anaesthetists
PRST	pressure, rate, sweating and tears
PVR	pulmonary vascular resistance
RBC	red blood cell
RMS	root mean square
RNA	ribonucleic acid
RR	respiratory rate
SBA	single best answer
SCID	severe combined immunodeficiency
SHO	senior house officer
SSRI	selective serotonin reuptake inhibitors
SV	stroke volume
SVP	saturated vapour pressure
SVR	systemic vascular resistance
SVT	supraventricular tachycardia
TCA	tricarboxylic acid
TOF	train of four
TURP	transurethral resection of the prostrate
Vd	volume of distribution
VF	ventricular fibrillation
VIC	vaporizer in circuit
VIE	vacuum insulated evaporator
VOC	vaporizer out of circuit
VT	ventricular tachycardia
WCC	white blood cell count

INTRODUCTION

The college has recently introduced single best answer (SBA) questions in addition to the multiple choice questions (MCQ) for the Primary FRCA examinations. The MCQ part of the Primary FRCA examination tests knowledge of the basic sciences needed in anaesthetic practice whereas assessment of 'knows how' and 'knows why' rather than simply 'knows' is better assessed by SBA questions.

The SBA questions are written by individual examiners, and then refined by an MCQ sub-group who agree on the single best answer using evidence from the published literature, standard texts or expert opinion, and consensus from the members of the examining board.

SBAs consist of a stem, lead-in question and five options. The stem is a vignette in clinical anaesthesia and its basic sciences. The stem has a maximum of 60 words focusing on a single problem. The lead-in is short and precise and poses a single question. The five options should all be possible solutions or responses to the question arising from the stem. However, one of the options will be the best response, and the remaining four will be inferior.

A useful approach for candidates is to read the stem and lead-in question while covering up the five options so that they cannot be seen. The answer that occurs to a well-prepared candidate at this stage, and then appears in the list of options, is likely to be the correct best response.

Candidates make a single mark on their answer sheet next to their choice for each question. Marks will only be awarded for a single correct answer. If candidates make more than one response to a question then no marks will be awarded for that question.

Further reading

Brennan, L. (2009). Single best answer MCQs. *RCoA Bulletin*, **57**, 39–41.

STRUCTURE AND MARKING OF MCQ/SBA PAPER

The Primary MCQ is blue printed to the Basic Level Curriculum. It is a written examination taken at various centres across the UK.

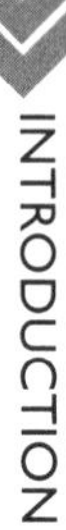

Structure of the exam

- 90 multiple choice questions in three hours, 60 × multiple true/false (MTF) questions plus 30 × single best answer (SBA) questions, comprising approximately of
  - 20 MTF question in pharmacology;
  - 20 MTF questions in physiology, including related biochemistry and anatomy;
  - 20 questions in physics, clinical measurement and data interpretation;
  - 30 SBA questions in any of the categories listed above.

The marking system

- One mark will be awarded for each correct answer in the MTF section.
- Four marks will be awarded for each correct question in the SBA section.
- The marks for each section are combined to produce a total mark.
- With 60 MTF and 30 SBA the maximum mark obtainable for the MCQ paper is 420 marks.
- The Pass mark is set by the examiners using Angoff Referencing. To allow for the examination's reliability this mark is then reduced by one standard error of measurement (SEM) to give the pass mark.
- Pass marks and scores are given in raw score and percentages.
- No marks deducted for incorrect answers.

Further reading

http://www.rcoa.ac.uk/primary-frca-mcq/structure-and-marking

PAPER 1 QUESTIONS

Question 1

During preparation for transfer of an intubated patient to the intensive care unit (ICU), it is noted that the pressure gauge on the size D oxygen cylinder reads 68.5 kPa. You have calculated the oxygen consumption to be 5 L per minute. How much time do you have to safely transfer the patient without the oxygen running out?

A. 12 minutes
B. 20 minutes
C. 34 minutes
D. 44 minutes
E. 68.5 minutes

Question 2

Initial pharmacotherapy for the patient with angina includes sublingual nitroglycerine. Relaxation of vascular smooth muscle by nitroglycerine is due to its metabolism to an intermediate that is similar in structure and activity to which of the following?

A. Nitrogen dioxide
B. Nitrous oxide
C. Nitric oxide
D. Cyanide
E. Thiocyanate

Question 3

You are asked to experimentally estimate total body water. Which single best technique would provide you with an estimate of this?

A. Inulin
B. Radioactively labelled carbon
C. Evan's blue dye
D. Use of deuterium isotope
E. Mannitol

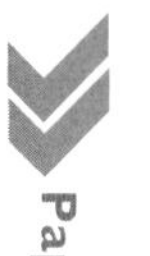

Question 4

In clinical trials, a new drug was found to reduce the risk of vasospasm after subarachnoid haemorrhage from 40% to 20%. What is the number needed to treat for this new drug?

A. 5
B. 10
C. 15
D. 20
E. 50

Question 5

A 47-year-old woman is admitted to the intensive care unit. She has taken a propranolol overdose and was found to be hypotensive and bradycardic. Her observations in the emergency department showed a blood pressure of 70/40 mm Hg and a heart rate of 34 beats per minute. After treatment with fluids, her blood pressure does not improve and she remains bradycardic. Which one of the following is most likely to improve the haemodynamics?

A. Atropine
B. Isoproterenol
C. Dopamine
D. Calcium
E. Glucagon

Question 6

You have requested blood components for a patient with a coagulopathy who has already undergone a massive transfusion. Which of the following statements best describes the correct information regarding blood products?

A. Blood consists of red blood cells and plasma.
B. Serum is a product of coagulated blood.
C. Plasma is synonymous with serum in clinical practice.
D. Immunoglobulins do not contribute to blood viscosity.
E. Fibrinogen, clotting factors and albumin are present in serum.

Question 7

A new test for detecting deep vein thrombosis has been developed. Out of 1000 people subjected to the test, 900 tested positive for the test and 800 of these were subsequently shown to have a thrombus. Of those who tested negative, 75 were subsequently shown to have a thrombus. Which of the following statements regarding the test is true?

A. The sensitivity of this test is 80%.
B. The sensitivity of this test is 90%.
C. The sensitivity of this test is 94%.
D. The specificity of this test is 20%.
E. The specificity of this test is 75%.

Question 8

A 30-year-old, 38-weeks pregnant, primigravid woman is scheduled to have an elective caesarean section for breech presentation and is seen by you in the antenatal clinic. She has a history of deep vein thrombosis, and the obstetric physician has adjusted her medications. The woman would like to know: which of the following drugs would not cross the placenta and would have no significant concentration in the milk on breastfeeding?

A. Heparin
B. Dicumarol
C. Warfarin
D. Phenindione
E. Acenocoumarol

Question 9

A 12-year-old African Caribbean boy with sickle cell disease is admitted to the accident and emergency department. He has a haemoglobin (Hb) level of 7 due to chronic anaemia with a high reticulocyte count. Which of the following statements is not true of red blood cells?

A. They derive from the myeloid stem cell lineage.
B. They derive from haemopoietic pluripotent stem cells.
C. Erythropoietin is produced by the liver and the kidney.
D. Vitamin B_{12} and folate are involved in DNA synthesis.
E. Reticulocytes are a product of red cell degradation.

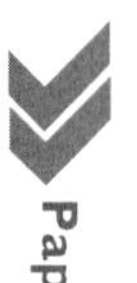

Question 10

During anaesthesia for foot surgery, core temperature is most accurately measured in which of the following areas?

A. Rectum
B. Bladder
C. Upper oesophagus
D. Axilla
E. Nasopharynx

Question 11

A 30-year-old patient was found unresponsive by his neighbour and has been admitted to the ICU. The admission findings read: comatose and unresponsive to pain, pupils dilated and not reacting to light, absent bowel sounds, dry oral mucosa, heart rate 150 beats per minute and blood pressure 104/55 mm Hg, with the electrocardiogram (ECG) showing right bundle branch block. These findings are suggestive of an overdose caused by which of the following?

A. Alprazolam
B. Lithium
C. Amitriptyline
D. Trazodone
E. Phenelzine

Question 12

A 78-year-old man is scheduled for repair of para-umbilical hernia. In your pre-operative assessment, you discover the patient has a polycythaemia. Which of the following statements does not support the pathophysiology of polycythaemia?

A. Polycythaemia increases blood viscosity.
B. Polycythaemia can be due to chronic hyperoxaemia.
C. Patients may develop heart failure as a consequence.
D. Polycythaemia can occur in burn patients.
E. Peri-operative risks include bleeding and thrombosis.

Question 13

While providing ventilation via an endotracheal tube, you suspect that there is turbulent flow. Which of the following strategies would be most appropriate to making the flow laminar?

A. Increasing the flow rate
B. Decreasing viscosity of the inspired gases
C. Cooling the inspired gases
D. Manipulating the parameters so that the Reynolds number is 500 kg/m/sec
E. Using a helium and oxygen mix

Question 14

An elderly man presents for pre-operative assessment. When asked about drug allergies, he indicates that he has none, but that he had significant effects on short- and long-term memory with a drug that was given to him during his last admission. The drug being described belongs to which of the following categories?

A. Phenothiazines
B. Tricyclic antidepressants
C. Benzodiazepines
D. MAO inhibitors
E. Butyrophenones

Question 15

A 40-year-old African Caribbean woman has an Hb level of 7.8 g/dL. She has a mean corpuscular volume (MCV) of 72 fL, platelets 170×10^9/L and white blood cell count (WCC) 6.8×10^9/L from blood results taken yesterday. She suffers from large menstrual losses. She is otherwise well and has no significant past medical history apart from having three normal vaginal deliveries at hospital in the UK. She is scheduled for an elective shoulder arthroscopy. Which of the following is most likely to be the cause of her anaemia?

A. Alcoholism
B. Bone marrow failure
C. Iron deficiency anaemia
D. Acute blood loss only
E. Sickle cell disease

Question 16

On the ICU, a new ultrasonic nebulization system has been introduced to humidify inspired gases. Which of the following considerations is most relevant in providing safe humidification when using this system?

A. As relative humidity above 80% is rarely generated, mucus plugs are likely to form.
B. Temperature must be monitored to prevent thermal injury to respiratory tissues.
C. Droplets with a size of 20 microns (μm) have the potential to cause pulmonary oedema.
D. Because of the destructive properties of ultrasound, it reduces the risk of cross-infection.
E. They have the potential to create turbulent flow within the breathing system.

Question 17

A diabetic patient presents with a cough associated with haemoptysis along with consistent fever (39°C). A chest X-ray shows left lobar pneumonia. Gram staining reveals Gram-positive diplococci. Correct therapy would be to administer which of the following?

A. Gentamicin
B. Penicillin G
C. Carbenicillin and gentamicin
D. Ampicillin
E. Ciprofloxacin

Question 18

A 65-year-old man is scheduled for repair of a right inguinal hernia. Review of blood results on your hospital's haematology electronic system shows he has a chronic anaemia of 7.4 g/dL. Which of the following are you most likely to find on examination and investigation of this patient?

A. Blood pressure 65/30 mmHg
B. A systolic murmur
C. Increased viscosity
D. Decreased cardiac output
E. Decreased 2,3-diphosphoglycerate (2,3-DPG)

Question 19

While providing anaesthesia for thyroid surgery, saturations are lower than expected, and the pulse oximeter trace is of good quality. A blood gas analysis is done and shows arterial blood gas (PaO_2) of 13 kPa. Past medical history includes chronic obstructive pulmonary disease (COPD) and liver cirrhosis. Which of the following is most likely to be the cause of the low pulse oximeter reading?

A. Diathermy.
B. Bilirubinaemia.
C. The patient is likely to a smoker.
D. Methylene blue infusion.
E. Sodium nitroprusside infusion.

Question 20

A severe asthmatic is being treated for respiratory distress. His weight is 60 kg, and the plasma theophylline concentration is 5 mg/L. The plan is to raise his plasma theophylline concentration from 5 mg/L to 15 mg/L to improve him clinically. A clearance value of 0.4 mL/min/kg is taken as the average value for theophylline, and if the volume of distribution (Vd) is 0.5 L/kg, then what would be the precise loading dose?

A. 900 mg
B. 600 mg
C. 300 mg
D. 1200 mg
E. 100 mg

Question 21

A patient is scheduled for a laparoscopic nephrectomy. A group and screen show that the patient's blood group is A rhesus negative. Which of the following is most appropriate to administer to this patient safely when needed?

A. Plasma serum containing anti-A
B. Red cell expressing the B antigen
C. Cryoprecipitate from any donor
D. Plasma from a B negative donor
E. Un-cross-matched platelets

Question 22

An American Society of Anesthesiologists (ASA) physical status 1 patient received a rapid sequence induction with 400 mg thiopentone and 100 mg suxamethonium during an emergency laparotomy for a perforated gastric ulcer. Further muscle relaxation was achieved with repeated doses of atracurium. At the end of the procedure, the 'train of four' test was used to assess residual neuromuscular blockade. Which of the following statements regarding the train of four test is most accurate?

A. The negative electrode should be placed proximally.
B. The train of four ratio is the force of the first twitch divided by the force of the last one.
C. The train of four ratio is typically 1 when suxamethonium is used.
D. The test is inaccurate if repeated within 2 minutes.
E. A supramaximal stimulus of 50 Amps is usually applied.

Question 23

An elderly woman with atrial fibrillation was commenced on warfarin. Warfarin will prevent clot formation in the left atrium. Which of the following statements most precisely describes the action of warfarin?

A. It partially inhibits synthesis of vitamin K–dependent clotting factors.
B. It inhibits synthesis of clotting factors in the spleen.
C. It inactivates precursors made active by γ-carboxylation of lysine acid residues.
D. It prevents reduction of the oxidized form of vitamin K.
E. It prevents the synthesis of vitamin K.

Question 24

A 28-year-old pregnant woman with known placenta praevia has undergone an emergency caesarean section for bleeding per vagina at 37 weeks. She required six units of blood and three units of fresh frozen plasma (FFP). Which of the following is least likely to be seen as a complication of a blood transfusion in this woman?

A. Delayed haemolytic reaction
B. Transfusion-related acute lung injury
C. Coagulopathy
D. Febrile transfusion reaction
E. Transmission of variant Creutzfeldt–Jakob disease (CJD)

Question 25

Which of the following best describes a circle breathing system?

A. Efficiency is increased when the adjustable pressure-limiting (APL) valve is downstream of the fresh gas flow.
B. The CO_2 absorber should be placed downstream of the reservoir bag.
C. The APL valve is usually found downstream of the reservoir bag.
D. Most systems incorporate a circle vaporizer.
E. Plenum vaporizers are favoured when the vaporizer is in circuit.

Question 26

Anaesthetic trainees attending a Royal College Primary FRCA revision course were being taught the subject of pharmacology. While discussing the concept of drug interactions, the teacher puts up a slide of an isobologram (see third figure below). The correct interpretation is which of the following?

A. Point A (½, ½) means synergism.
B. Point B (½, ¼) means additivity.
C. Point C (½, ¾) means antagonism.
D. A line from 1 on the X axis to 1 on the Y axis means synergism.
E. A line from 1 on the X axis to 1 on the Y axis means potentiation.

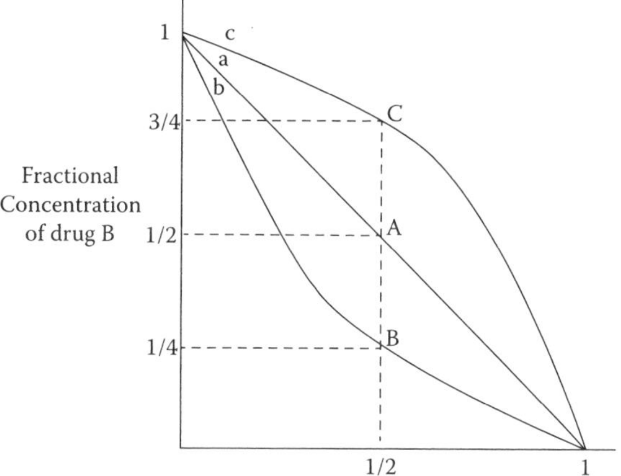

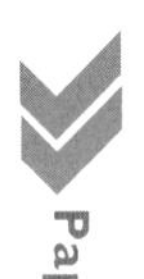

Question 27

An 18-year-old female presents to the preoperative clinic and gives a history of having had a haematopoietic stem cell transplant. Her sister died at a young age from the same disorder, having acquired severe pneumonia. Which of the following is the most likely reason for her stem cell transplant?

A. HIV/AIDS
B. Organ transplant
C. Neutropaenia following 5-flourouracil
D. Steroid use
E. Severe combined immunodeficiency

Question 28

While working with the military, you are required to administer anaesthesia for retrieving shrapnel from a soldier. The only available vaporizer is an Oxford miniature vaporizer (OMV). Isoflurane, sevoflurane and halothane are available. Oxygen and air cylinders are also available. Which of the following would most increase the safety profile when using the OMV?

A. Avoid muscle relaxation, and allow the patient to breathe spontaneously if possible.
B. Connect the vaporizer to compressed gas to improve vapour performance and to maintain constant output.
C. The Oxford miniature vaporizer should ideally be used with halothane, as it was originally calibrated with halothane.
D. Ventilation is preferred as the vaporizer has a high intrinsic resistance which increases the work of breathing.
E. The lack of temperature compensation mechanisms will require vigilance to maintain adequate doses.

Question 29

Anaesthetic trainees attending a Royal College Primary FRCA revision course were being taught the subject of pharmacology. The Vaughan–Williams classification of antiarrhythmic is best matched by which of the following combinations?

A. Quinidine = shortens the refractory period of cardiac muscle
B. Lignocaine = prolongs the refractory period of cardiac muscle
C. Flecainide = no effect on the refractory period of cardiac muscle
D. Verapramil = $K+$ channel blockade
E. Sotalol = B receptor blockade

Question 30

A 37-year-old woman is scheduled for an emergency explorative laparotomy for abdominal pain and worsening metabolic acidosis. She tells you she has recently undergone investigations for a bleeding disorder. She is due to meet the Consultant Haematologist next week for a diagnosis. Which of the following is she least likely to have?

A. Thrombocytopaenia purpura
B. von Willebrand disease
C. Haemophilia B
D. Factor V Leiden
E. Disseminated intravascular coagulation

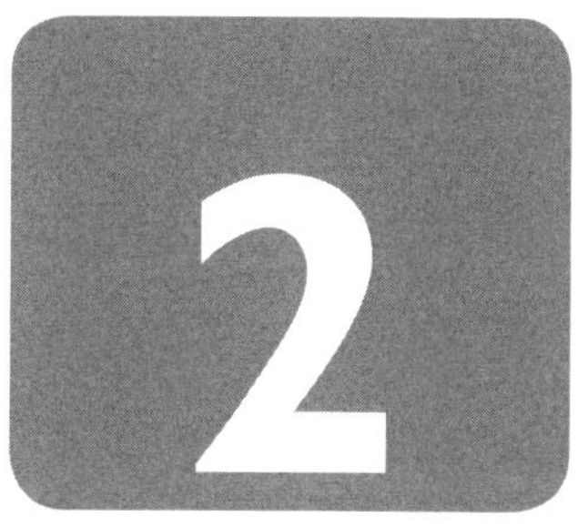

PAPER 1 ANSWERS

Answer 1: C

Oxygen cylinders contain compressed gas. The size D oxygen cylinder contains 340 L of oxygen when filled to a pressure of 137 kPa. Boyle's law states that at constant temperature, volume is inversely proportional to the pressure. Hence, at 68.5 kPa:

$$\begin{aligned} \text{Remaining volume} &= 68.5\ \text{kPa} / 137\ \text{kPa} \times 340\ \text{L} \\ &= 0.5 \times 340\ \text{L} \\ &= 170\ \text{L} \end{aligned}$$

At an oxygen consumption of 5 L/min, the time remaining before exhaustion of the cylinder is

$$170\ \text{L} / 5\ \text{L} / \text{min} = 34\ \text{min}$$

Size C and D cylinders hold 170 and 680 L respectively when filled to a pressure of 137 kPa.

Further reading

BOC Healthcare. Medical gas cylinder data chart. 2009. http://www.bochealthcare.co.uk/images/local/content_pages/safety/cylinder_chart/cylinder_data_chart.pdf

Davey, A., and Diba, A. *Ward's Anaesthetic Equipment*. 5th ed. London: Elsevier Saunders, 2005.

Answer 2: C

Though the exact mechanism by which nitroglycerine (glyceryl trinitrate [GTN]) produces vasodilation is not completely understood, it is thought that GTN is metabolized by denitration to form nitric oxide. Nitric oxide is an endogenous endothelial-derived relaxing factor, and is known to be a potent vasodilator. *In vivo*, nitric oxide is derived from the metabolism of L-arginine and is synthesized in the endothelium. Once it is synthesized, it rapidly diffuses into myocytes to induce relaxation by the activation of the guanylate cyclase pathway.

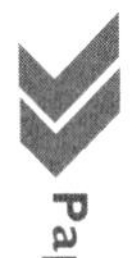

Further reading

Peck, T.E., Williams, M., and Hill, S.A. *Pharmacology for Anaesthesia and Intensive Care*. Cambridge: Cambridge University Press, 2003.

Answer 3: D

Total body water in the adult can be estimated as being 60% of body weight in Kg. This water is distributed in two main body compartments – the extracellular fluid (ECF) compartment and the intracellular fluid (ICF) compartment. The ratio of these compartments is roughly 1:2 ECF:ICF. The ECF encompasses the interstitial and plasma fluid compartments as well as the transcellular fluid (cerebrospinal, pleural, peritoneal, synovial, aqueous and bile fluids). The ICF compartment is a combination of plasma fluid and blood cell volume.

The volumes of each compartment can be experimentally calculated by measuring the concentrations of known quantities of the various tracers that are known to be confined to a particular fluid compartment and that are neither excreted nor metabolized by using the equation:

Volume of compartment = mass of tracer administered to compartment / concentration of tracer measured in compartment

Below is a list of some tracers used to measure particular compartments:

- Total body water: isotopic water
- ECF: Mannitol and inulin
- Blood: isotopic red cells
- Plasma: tracer-labelled albumin and Evan's blue dye

Further reading

Spoors, C., and Kiff, K. *Training in Anaesthesia: The Essential Curriculum*. Oxford: Oxford University Press, 2010, 291.

Answer 4: A

The number needed to treat (NNT) is the number of patients needed to be treated to avoid one additional bad outcome. NNT is calculated as follows:

NNT = 1 / Absolute risk reduction

The absolute risk reduction for this example is 0.40 – 0.20 = 0.2 (20%). Therefore, the NNT for the new drug is 1 / 0.2 = 5.

Further reading

Centre for Evidence Based Medicine. Number needed to treat. http://www.cebm.net/index.aspx?o=1044

Yentis, S., Hirsch, N., and Smith, G. *Anaesthesia and Intensive Care A–Z*. 4th ed. London: Churchill Livingstone, 2009.

Answer 5: E

β-blockers work by blocking cardiovascular receptors in both the cardiac and vascular muscle. Its central action on the heart is bradycardia and reduced contractility, while they cause peripheral vasodilatation. Both of these actions would produce a combined effect of bradycardia with hypotension. The antidote for β-blocker toxicity is glucagon, as this improves ionotropy. The dose of glucagon is 3 mg of intravenous (IV) glucagon initially followed by an infusion (if needed) until all the cardiovascular effects of propranolol have reversed. Electrolyte correction with calcium and potassium is not the primary treatment for β-blocker toxicity. Dopamine, isoprenaline and adrenaline may not occur as frequently as glucagon in β-blocker overdose as these agents would require free β adrenergic receptors.

Further reading

Peck, T.E., Williams, M., and Hill, S.A. *Pharmacology for Anaesthesia and Intensive Care*. Cambridge: Cambridge University Press, 2003.

Answer 6: B

Blood consists of red blood cells, white blood cells, platelets and a liquid called *plasma*. When uncoagulated whole blood is centrifuged, it separates into its cellular components (at the bottom) and a fluid phase (at the top). This fluid phase is referred to as plasma and contains proteins (including albumin, immunoglobulins, clotting factors and fibrinogen), nutrients (glucose and amino acids), hormones, ions and water. When whole blood is coagulated, the fluid component that is left is called *serum* and is similar in composition to plasma, but is devoid of clotting factors.

Answer 7: D

The sensitivity of a test is the ability to identify true positives. This is given by the following:

$$\text{Sensitivity} = \text{true positives} / (\text{true positives} + \text{false negatives})$$

In this example:

$$\text{Sensitivity} = 800 / (800 + 75) = 91.4\%$$

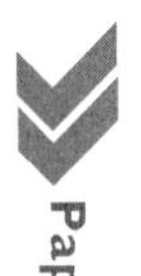
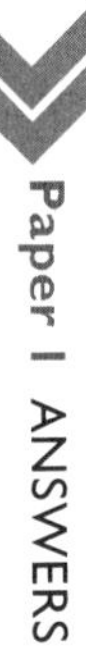

The specificity of the test is the property of the test to be able to correctly identify those without the disease. It is determined by this equation:

Specificity = true negatives / (true negatives + false positives)

Using the same example:

Specificity = 25 / (25 + 100) = 20%

Further reading

Lalkhen, A.G., and McCluskey, A. Clinical tests: sensitivity and specificity. *Contin Educ Anaesth Crit Care Pain* (2008) 8 (6): 221–3.

Answer 8: A

Heparin, being a large molecule, does not cross the placenta easily. It is a polymer, consisting of 8–15 disaccharide units. Furthermore, heparin given to the mother is not secreted into breast milk. Thus, breastfeeding is safe for the baby. Despite these benefits of heparin, the rate of haemorrhage or stillbirths in pregnant anticoagulated patients is not dissimilar to that of similar patients anticoagulated with warfarin.

Further reading

Peck, T.E., Williams, M., and Hill, S.A. *Pharmacology for Anaesthesia and Intensive Care*. Cambridge: Cambridge University Press, 2003.

Answer 9: E

Red blood cells derive from the myeloid lineage of the haemopoeitic pluripotent stem cell. Red blood cells, also called *erythroblasts*, start their life as proerythroblasts that contain nuclear material (DNA). These cells mature in the bone marrow, and as they do so they synthesize haemoglobin. The DNA contained in the nucleus is eventually expelled from the cell. The proerythrocyte has now become a reticulocyte and enters the circulation from the bone marrow. Further maturation takes place in the circulation over 1–2 days, and the remaining RNA is lost to leave a mature red blood cell, an erythrocyte which is anucleate. Iron is essential for haemoglobin production. Vitamin B_{12} and folate are nutrients essential for the synthesis of nucleic acids, which are the building blocks of DNA. Lack of B_{12} and folate causes reduced DNA synthesis and a macrocytic anaemia where cells have a reduced life span. Red cells are destroyed by the reticulo-endothelial system by phagocytosis.

Further reading

Power, I., and Kam, P. *Principles of Physiology for the Anaesthetist*. 2nd ed. London: Hodder Arnold, 2008, 269–7.

Answer 10: E

Core temperature is defined as the temperature of the blood perfusing vital organs such as the brain. Variations of temperature exist between body sites because of regional blood flow differences and because of increased heat loss in particular areas. Measurement in the lower oesophagus, the nasopharynx, and the blood using a Swan–Ganz catheter most accurately reflect the core temperature. Temperature measurement in the rectum may be inaccurate because of insulation from faeces, and because of the cooling effects of blood returning from the lower limbs. The bladder temperature is dependent on the flow of urine, and high flows are necessary to ensure accurate measurement of core temperature. Probes placed behind the soft palate give good approximations of the core temperature. However, if incorrectly placed, they are prone to inaccuracies because of the flow of inspired gases. Tympanic temperature has also been shown to mirror core temperature. However, if the probe is not correctly placed or if wax is present, inaccurate readings are likely.

Further reading

Anaesthesia UK. 2005. Temperature measurement sites. http://www.frca.co.uk/article.aspx?articleid=100352

Rao, S., and Rajan, M. 2008. Heat production and loss: update in anaesthesia. http://update.anaesthesiologists.org/wp-content/uploads/2008/12/Heat-Production-and-Loss.pdf

Answer 11: C

The overdose effects of various drugs are as follows:

- Alprazolam: a benzodiazepine analogue that would produce central effects (coma) but minimal cardiac or anticholinergic effects
- Amitriptyline: coma, tachycardia, prolonged QRS duration on electrocardiogram (ECG), and anticholinergic signs
- Lithium: will produce coma with bradyarrhythmias but no anticholinergic effects
- Phenelzine: a MAO inhibitor that will produce sympathomimetic effects like hypertension, tachycardia, hyperthermia and sweating
- Trazodone: a non-tricyclic antidepressant; may cause hypotension due to its alpha blockade but has no anticholinergic effects

Further reading

Peck, T.E., Williams, M., and Hill, S.A. *Pharmacology for Anaesthesia and Intensive Care*. Cambridge: Cambridge University Press, 2003.

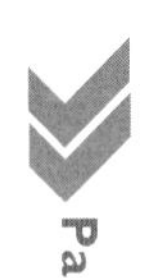

Answer 12: B

Polycythaemia is a condition characterized by elevated haemoglobin concentration, usually >16–17 g/dL, or a greater than normal red cell count or haematocrit. Causes may be due to primary bone marrow pathology (polycythaemia rubra vera), iatrogenic (over-transfusion or over-treatment with erythropoietin), secondary to chronic hypoxic drive (those with chronic obstructive pulmonary disease [COPD] and smokers) and as an adaptation to living at high altitude. Polycythaemia can also be relative (i.e. relative loss of plasma volume as seen in burns patients or those who are extremely intravascularly dehydrated). Clinical manifestations are due to hyperviscosity and, in some cases, hypervolaemia (headaches, visual disturbance, cardiac failure due to decreased cardiac output and thrombotic phenomena) and a high rate of metabolism (sweating and loss of weight). These patients are also at risk of bleeding due to a relative dilution of platelets and coagulation factors.

Further reading

Yentis, S., Hirsch, N., and Smith, G. *Anaesthesia and Intensive Care A–Z*. 4th ed. London: Churchill Livingstone, 2009.

Answer 13: E

Turbulent flow occurs when the Reynolds number is in excess of 2000. The Reynolds number is calculated by the following equation:

$$Re = \frac{\rho VD}{\mu}$$

where:

μ = the viscosity of the fluid;
V = the velocity of the object;
D = the diameter or length (basically, the shape of the object);
ρ = the density of the fluid.

The above equation can be manipulated to change turbulent flow, for example in upper-airway obstruction, to laminar flow. Laminar flow ensures more flow of gases through a tube as resistance to flow is reduced, and in airway obstruction it allows more oxygen to enter; furthermore, it reduces the work of breathing. Heliox, a mixture of helium and oxygen, is available in a 50/50 mix or a 20% oxygen and 80% helium mix. It reduces the work of breathing by shifting turbulent flow to laminar flow. This is achieved as Heliox has a lower density than air; 0.5 g/L versus 1.5 g/L at standard temperature and pressure.

Further reading

Davey, A., and Diba, A. *Ward's Anaesthetic Equipment*. 5th ed. London: Elsevier Saunders, 2005.

Answer 14: C

The vignette signifies the effects that a drug can have on memory. Benzodiazepines can affect a patient's short- and long-term memory, Furthermore, they also decrease attention span in cognitively impaired patients, thus worsening function. Despite this, benzodiazepines are often used to sedate patients with cognitive impairment.

Phenothiazines like some antidepressants can produce sedation but have not yet been proven to affect memory.

Further reading

Peck, T.E., Williams, M., and Hill, S.A. *Pharmacology for Anaesthesia and Intensive Care*. Cambridge: Cambridge University Press, 2003.

Answer 15: C

Anaemia can be classified into macrocytic, microcytic and normocytic depending on whether the mean cell volume is high, low or normal, respectively. An alternative strategy is to classify anaemia as acute or chronic. This woman has a microcytic anaemia. Causes include iron deficiency, which may be due to increased requirements (e.g. pregnancy), increased loss (e.g. chronic bleeding), decreased iron intake (e.g. malnutrition) or anaemia of chronic disease. A macrocytic anaemia is seen with B_{12}–folate deficiencies, alcoholism, hypothyroidism, pregnancy (dilutional anaemia with macrocytosis and/or also due to B_{12}–folate deficiency) and bone marrow infiltration. Normocytic anaemias can be seen with acute blood loss, haemolytic diseases (sickle cell disease, auto-immune etc.), chronic renal and liver disease and bone marrow failure. Sometimes, the picture is mixed and clinical judgement needs to be exercised. This woman is unlikely to have sickle cell disease as she has remained asymptomatic up until now. Acute blood loss would not cause a drop in mean corpuscular volume so quickly, and the other options are usually accompanied by a macrocytosis.

Further reading

Raftery, A.T., and Lim, E. *Churchill's Pocketbook of Differential Diagnosis*. Edinburgh: Churchill Livingstone, 2001, 24–8.

Answer 16: E

Droplets are generated when water comes into contact with the vibrating surface of the ultrasonic nebulizer. The vibrations are usually in the range of a few megahertz. Droplets of varying sizes can be generated, and those with a diameter of 1 micron (μm) easily reach the alveoli. Droplets of greater size are deposited in the upper respiratory tract or breathing system (20 μm), or are deposited in the trachea (5 μm). A large amount of water can be nebulized into the gas, which if deposited in the alveoli can result in pulmonary oedema. Small-diameter droplets

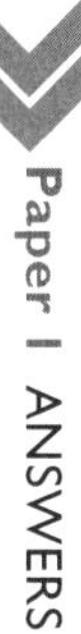

are very stable and can carry infection readily. As more water is added to the inspired gases, the density of the gas increases, hence increasing the Reynolds number and propensity to turbulent flow.

Further reading

Davies, P., and Kenny, G. *Basic Physics and Measurement in Anaesthesia*. 5th ed. London: Butterworth Heinemann, 2005.

Answer 17: B

Diabetic patients are more susceptible to infections. This patient has a pneumonic patch on the left lung. Penicillin G is the drug of choice for Gram-positive diplococci (pneumococcal pneumonia). Gentamycin can be used, but it is most effective on Gram-negative organisms. Other drugs that can be used are carbenicillin and ampicillin; however, they are not first-line. Ciproflaxacin is only moderately active against streptococci species.

Further reading

Peck, T.E., Williams, M., and Hill, S.A. *Pharmacology for Anaesthesia and Intensive Care*. Cambridge: Cambridge University Press, 2003.

Answer 18: B

Haemoglobin concentration is a major determinant of the oxygen-carrying capacity and content of blood. Anaemia reduces this, resulting in symptoms of fatigue, lethargy and breathlessness, and at extremes can compromise coronary oxygen delivery and result in angina. There is a relative increase in plasma volume (to maintain circulating volume). This results in a decreased viscosity which increases and improves flow up until a critical level, after which oxygen delivery is compromised causing anaemic hypoxia. Decreased oxygen carrying capacity causes a compensatory increase in cardiac output, and a flow murmur is often heard on auscultation of the chest. 2,3-diphosphoglycerate (2,3-DPG) levels are increased. An acute anaemia from haemorrhagic loss is likely to cause hypotension, but this is unlikely to be seen in the chronic setting as there is time for the body to adapt physiologically.

Further reading

Yentis, S., Hirsch, N., and Smith, G. *Anaesthesia and Intensive Care A–Z*. 4th ed. London: Churchill Livingstone, 2009.

Answer 19: D

The accuracy of pulse oximetry can be affected by low perfusion states (e.g. vasoconstriction, hypothermia, hypotension and cardiac arrest) where the pulsatile component is too small to process into a meaningful result. Furthermore, interference from diathermy, motion artefacts (e.g. shivering) and ambient light are known to reduce data quality. Methaemoglobinaemia generated from nitrates (sodium nitroprusside) and local anaesthetics produce an under-reading of saturations, as methaemoglobin absorbs maximally at the same wavelength as deoxygenated haemoglobin (660 nm). Methylene blue and indocyanine dyes also generate inaccurately low readings. In thyroid surgery, methylene blue is often infused to identify the parathyroids and is likely to be the reason for low saturations. There is no indication of the administration of sodium nitroprusside in this scenario. Smokers may have a high level of carboxyhaemoglobin (10–15%) and hence overestimates of saturation are possible. Bilirubin does not absorb at the wavelengths employed by the pulse oximeter.

Further reading

Jubran, A. Pulse oximetry. *Crit Care* (1999) 3: R11–R17.

Answer 20: C

The equation to be applied here is

$$D = Vd \times Cp$$

where:

D = total amount of drug in body;
Vd = volume of distribution; and
Cp = plasma concentration.

Vd is expressed as L/kg.

Thus, in this patient the Vd would be 30 L (60 kg × 0.5 L/kg). At a concentration of 15 mg/L, there should be 450 mg of theophylline in his body (15 mg/L × 30 L). Prior to the loading dose, his body contains 150 mg of the drug (5 mg/L × 30 L). In order to shift the plasma concentration from 5 to 15 mg/L, the new loading dose to be given would be 300 mg (150–450 mg). The clearance value would not be needed to calculate the loading dose as per this equation.

Further reading

Peck, T.E., Williams, M., and Hill, S.A. *Pharmacology for Anaesthesia and Intensive Care*. Cambridge: Cambridge University Press, 2003.

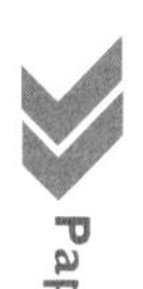

Answer 21: C

Red cells can express a variety of antigens – ABO, rhesus and Kell, to name a few. The commonest and most clinically significant ones are the ABO group and the rhesus group.

Patients with blood group A express antigen A and carry an antibody to antigen B in their plasma. Those with blood group B express antigen B and carry an anti-A antibody. Patients with blood group AB red cells express both A and B antigens and have no antibodies in their plasma (universal recipient). Patients with blood group O express no antigens on their RBC surface and carry anti-A and anti-B antibodies in their plasma (universal donors). ABO antibodies arise naturally without previous contact with an antigen.

Plasma is that component of whole blood which is obtained from removal of all cellular components and contains clotting factors, fibrinogen, water, salts, proteins such as albumin, immunoglobulins and so on.

Fresh frozen plasma is derived from plasma and contains albumin, the majority of the clotting factors, and very little if any fibrinogen as this is precipitated to derive cryoprecipitate (also rich in Factor 8 and von Willebrand factor).

Potentially life-threatening reactions can occur as a result of incorrect administration of blood products to patients – such as donor cells reacting with recipient plasma or donor plasma reacting with recipient cells.

In a group and screen test, red cells are ABO typed and the serum is tested to identify any other atypical antibodies. During cross-matching, donor cells are mixed with patient serum to identify any reactions before the blood product is deemed compatible for transfusion. Donor blood is screened for atypical antibodies, and so donor plasma usually need not be tested with recipient cells. These processes help to identify ABO and other blood group incompatibilities.

The other group which is important in blood product cross-matching and blood typing is rhesus. An individual is rhesus-positive if he or she carries the D antigen. Antibodies are formed on exposure to the rhesus antigen in naïve patients. These are immunoglobulin G (IgG) antibodies, and in women they can therefore can cross the placenta and cross-react with foetal red cells. For further information, please refer to the reference given here.

Further reading

Spoors, C., and Kiff, K. *Training in Anaesthesia: The Essential Curriculum*. Oxford: Oxford University Press, 2010, 384–5.

Answer 22: C

A supramaximal current (20–60 mAmps), is normally applied to ensure complete depolarization of the nerve. To minimize the current, the positive electrode is placed proximally. Four pulses are applied at a frequency of 2 Hz. and the train of four (TOF) ratio is the force of the fourth twitch to the force of the first. Fade is a feature of non-depolarizing neuromuscular blocking agents, and successive disappearance of twitches correlates with the percentage receptor blockade as follows:

Loss of Twitch	Percentage Receptor Blockade
4th	75%
3rd	80%
2nd	80%
1st	100%

The TOF ratio should be 0.9 to be adequately reversed. Administration of neostigmine to the reverse blockade should not be done if fewer than three twitches are observed.

Fade is not a feature of depolarizing neuromuscular blockers. Although the twitch height is reduced, the TOF ratio remains 1.0. The TOF can be repeated every 15 seconds without fear of inaccuracies.

Further reading

Conor, D., McGrath, C., and Hunter, J.M. Monitoring of neuromuscular block. *Contin Educ Anaesth Crit Care Pain* (2006) 6 (1): 7–12.

Yentis, S., Hirsch, N., and Smith, G. *Anaesthesia and Intensive Care A–Z*. 4th ed. London: Churchill Livingstone, 2009.

Answer 23: D

Warfarin exhibits its anticoagulant property by preventing the recycling of reduced vitamin K to the oxidized form. Oxidized vitamin K is required to mature precursors of clotting factors (II, VII, IX and X) by γ-carboxylation of glutamic acid residues. Warfarin takes up to 72 hours to exert its full effect.

Further reading

Peck, T.E., Williams, M., and Hill, S.A. *Pharmacology for Anaesthesia and Intensive Care*. Cambridge: Cambridge University Press, 2003.

Answer 24: E

Complications of blood transfusion can be classified into the following groups:

1. Immunity and incompatibility reactions: ABO, rhesus and other blood group haemolytic reactions – may be acute or delayed
2. Febrile reactions: non-haemolytic
3. Hypersensitivity reactions: rashes
4. Risk of infection: bacterial, viral (hepatitis, cytomegalovirus [CMV] and human immunodeficiency virus [HIV]), fungal and prion diseases
5. Biochemical disturbances: hyperkalaemia, hypocalcaemia, iron overload and metabolic acidosis

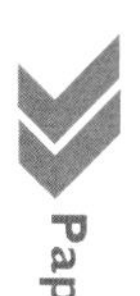

6. Haematological: dilutional coagulopathies, disseminated intravascular coagulation (DIC) and polycythaemia
7. Cardiac: fluid overload and cardiac failure
8. Respiratory: pulmonary oedema and transfusion-related acute lung injury
9. Other: hypothermia and shift of oxygen dissociation curve to the left

The risk of variant Creutzfeldt–Jakob disease (CJD) transmission is thought to be the least common of all risks.

Further reading

Maxwell, M.J., and Wilson, M.J.A. Complications of blood transfusion. *Contin Educ Anaesth Crit Care Pain* (2006) 6 (6): 225–9.
Spoors, C., and Kiff, K. *Training in Anaesthesia: The Essential Curriculum.* Oxford: Oxford University Press, 2010, 291.
Tranfusion Guidelines. http://www.transfusionguidelines.org.uk

Answer 25: B

The circle system consists of two one-way valves (V), a soda lime canister (S), a fresh gas flow (FGF), a reservoir bag (R) and an adjustable pressure-limiting (APL) valve. Excess gas exits via the APL valve before passing through the CO_2 absorber, and hence efficiency is improved. FGF enters downstream and is not wasted via the APL. Vaporizers may be in circuit (VICs) or out of circuit (VOCs), although most circle systems incorporate a plenum VOC. Plenum vaporizers with a high resistance are not suitable for VICs. Low-resistance vaporizers such as the Goldman are employed when VICs are necessary.

Further reading

Yentis, S., Hirsch, N., and Smith, G. *Anaesthesia and Intensive Care A–Z.* 4th ed. London: Churchill Livingstone, 2009.

Answer 26: C

An isobologram is used to study drug interactions. It graphically describes the combined effect of two drugs. In the scenario of these two drugs A and B, their fractional concentrations of a and b mmol/L are represented on X and Y axes, respectively. The points that will be produced by varying the fractional concentration of Drug B against a fixed concentration of Drug A in this scenario would be as follows:

Purely additive effect = straight line from 1 on the X axis (Drug A) to 1 on the Y axis (Drug B)

Point A (½, ½) = on the straight line indicates additivity

Point B (½, ¼) = on the concave line is synergism between drug A and B

C, (½, ¾) = on the convex line is antagonism between the two drugs

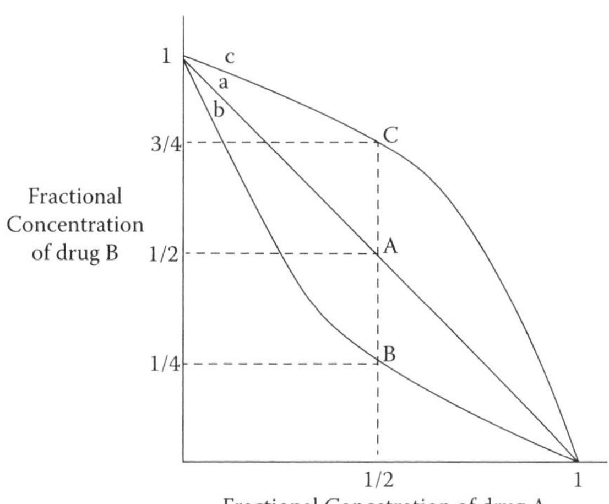

Further reading

Peck, T.E., Williams, M., and Hill, S.A. *Pharmacology for Anaesthesia and Intensive Care*. Cambridge: Cambridge University Press, 2003.

Answer 27: E

Peri-operative immunodeficiency is a major risk factor for surgical site infection. The causes can be divided into congenital and acquired. Congenital causes are rare and include severe combined immunodeficiency (SCID). Acquired causes are more common and include HIV/AIDS; diabetes (especially if poorly controlled); immunosuppressive therapies such as chemotherapy and radiotherapy; and drugs such as steroids, methotrexate, azathoprine and those used for organ transplant recipients, burns, trauma, splenectomy and connective tissue disorders.

Further reading

Schwartz, R.A. Pediatric severe combined immunodeficiency. http://emedicine.medscape.com/article/888072-overview

Yentis, S., Hirsch, N., and Smith, G. *Anaesthesia and Intensive Care A–Z*. 4th ed. London: Churchill Livingstone, 2009.

Answer 28: A

Draw-over vaporizers are incorporated directly into the breathing system, and the inspiratory effort of the patient draws gas through them. The system has an intrinsic low resistance to gas flow to minimize the work of breathing. Gas flowing into the vaporizer is split into two streams. One stream passes through the vaporizer and becomes saturated with the volatile agent. The other stream bypasses the vaporizer. Both streams converge distally, and this gas flows to the patient. The output of the vaporizer is dependent on the splitting ratio of the two streams,

which in turn is governed by a dial. Cooling of the vapour chamber occurs as a result of loss of energy from the latent heat of the vaporization, and output reduces at a set concentration over time (saturated vapour pressure is dependent on temperature). Temperature compensation mechanisms are frequently employed to maintain constant output. During spontaneous breathing, respiratory depression occurs with increasing volatile concentration. This automatically reduces the amount of gas passing through the vaporizer, and hence dangerous concentrations of volatile are not delivered. During positive pressure ventilation, however, this safety mechanism is absent. The Oxford miniature vaporizer can be used with halothane, isoflurane and trichloroethylene.

Further reading

Kamm, G., and Wilson, I.H. Draw-over anaesthesia part 1 – theory. *Update Anaesthes* (1992) (1): Article 3.

Davey, A., and Diba, A. *Ward's Anaesthetic Equipment*. 5th ed. London: Elsevier Saunders, 2005.

Answer 29: C

In the Vaughan–Williams classification of drugs, the sodium channel blockers which prolong the action potential are quinidine and procainamide (Class IA). Lignocaine, mexiletine and phenytoin are Class IB drugs and shorten action potential, while flecainide (Class IC) has no effect on the action potential.

Beta blockers are Class II drugs.

Sotalol (Class III) is a potassium channel blocker, while verapramil and diltiazem block calcium channels and are Class IV drugs.

Further reading

Peck, T.E., Williams, M., and Hill, S.A. *Pharmacology for Anaesthesia and Intensive Care*. Cambridge: Cambridge University Press, 2003.

Answer 30: D

Factor V Leiden and protein C or S deficiencies are inherited thrombophilia and result in a prothrombotic state. Thrombocytopaenia results in low platelets which can cause a tendency to bleed. Bleeding tendencies may also result from platelet dysfunction, hepatic failure, anticoagulation (due to warfarin, heparin etc.), haemophilia A and B (clotting Factor 8 and 9 deficiency, respectively) or von Willebrand disease (deficiency of von Willebrand factor – this factor is needed for the stability of Factor 8 and in the initial phase of platelet aggregation). DIC is a possibility in this case as the woman is suffering from an acute abdomen pain of unknown cause.

Further reading

Aitkenhead, A.R., Smith G., et al. *Textbook of Anaesthesia*. 5th ed. London: Churchill Livingstone Elsevier, 2007, 431–43.

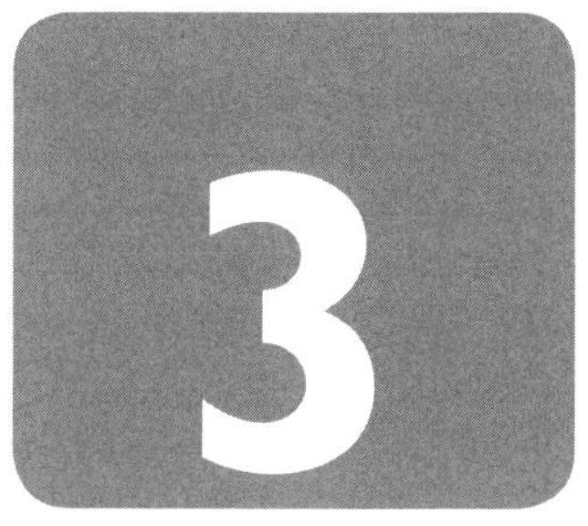

PAPER 2 QUESTIONS

Question 1

Which of the following best describes the anatomy and function of a Bain breathing system?

A. It is classified as a coaxial Mapleson B breathing system.
B. A carbon dioxide absorber is placed distal to the reservoir.
C. It incorporates two unidirectional valves placed on either side of the patient port.
D. It is more efficient during controlled ventilation than spontaneous ventilation.
E. It has a high internal resistance, making it unsuitable for spontaneous ventilation.

Question 2

A 70-year-old, 70 kg, previously well man was admitted on the stroke ward for left-sided arm and leg weakness. His carotid duplex scan showed a right internal carotid artery stenosis, and the vascular surgeon has scheduled him for a right carotid endarterectomy under a cervical plexus block. If he develops systemic local anaesthetic toxicity, his therapeutic intralipid (20%) dosing regime would be best described by which of the following statements?

A. Give an initial intravenous bolus of 10 mL 20% lipid emulsion over 1 min.
B. Start an immediate intravenous infusion of 20% intralipid at 1000 mL/hr.
C. At 5 min intervals, give two repeat boluses of 10 mL.
D. If no improvement after 5 min, increase the infusion rate to 3000 mL/hr.
E. Do not exceed a maximum cumulative dose of 1840 mL.

Question 3

A neurophysiologist is performing nerve conduction studies. Which of the following is not involved in the generation and propagation of an action potential?

A. Any magnitude of stimulus
B. The myelination of axons
C. Positive feedback mechanisms
D. Voltage gated ion channels
E. Saltatory conduction

Question 4

Choose the most correct statement regarding the Severinghaus electrode.

A. It does not require a power source.
B. The response time is typically 2 minutes.
C. The buffer is silver chloride.
D. The incorporated plastic membrane acts as a catalyst.
E. It can accurately measure oxygen tensions to within 0.001 kPa.

Question 5

Which of the following statements about ketorolac tromethamine is not true?

A. 10 mg of ketorolac has the analgesic equivalent of 50 mg pethidine.
B. 10 mg of ketorolac has the analgesic equivalent of 6 mg of morphine.
C. Ketorolac is a cyclooxygenase inhibitor which has a half-life of 3 hours.
D. Bronchospasm is a contraindication for the use of ketorolac.
E. Ketorolac may inhibit platelet aggregation and prolong bleeding time.

Question 6

A 35-year-old woman experiences extreme nausea post-operatively. She has received cyclizine, ondansetron, metoclorpramide, propofol and adequate fluid hydration. Which of the following receptors is most likely to be responsible for her nausea?

A. Histamine receptor
B. Alpha adrenoceptor
C. Muscarinic acetylcholine (ACH) receptor
D. Serotonin receptor
E. Beta 1 adrenoceptor

Question 7

You have performed a blood:gas analysis of an arterial sample. Which of the following is a derived value?

A. Bicarbonate concentration
B. PaO_2
C. $PaCO_2$
D. pH
E. Haemoglobin concentration

Question 8

A 28-year-old man was admitted to the psychiatric ward due to concerns he raised against his neighbours. He states that his neighbours had been spying on him and are now planning on killing him. He says that they had placed cameras in his house to monitor his activities. Last night, he heard them through the walls threatening to kill him. In order to protect himself, he has bought a gun. Which of the following drug is the best treatment for this behaviour?

A. Benztropine
B. Diazepam
C. Fluoxetine
D. Lithium
E. Risperidone

Question 9

A 63-year-old man diagnosed with an obstructive gastric malignancy has undergone a radical gastrectomy. Regarding gastric function, which of the following statements is incorrectly paired?

A. The gastric mucosa – is involved in the production of HCl at 0.15 M
B. Chief cells – produce intrinsic factor which is essential for absorption of vitamin B_{12}
C. Gastric acid – production is stimulated by gastrin
D. Pepsin – involved in proteolysis
E. Vagal stimuli – are involved in gastric mucus production

Question 10

A 45-year-old man requires inotropic support in intensive care to improve myocardial contractility. Which of the following statements regarding cardiac muscle contraction is false?

A. Cardiac muscle consists of striated muscle fibres connected into a syncytium.
B. Calcium is essential for cardiac muscle contraction.
C. The force of myocyte contraction is proportional to the intracellular calcium concentration.
D. Voltage-dependent sodium channels are involved in phase 0 of the cardiac myocyte contraction.
E. Repolarization of the cardiac myocyte is via inward K ion movement.

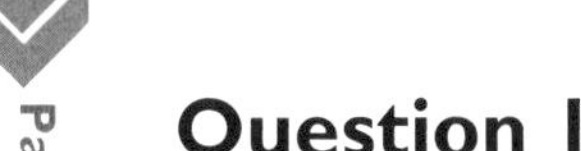

Question 11

A neonate born by emergency caesarean section 2 hours ago has pulse oximetry readings of 98% on the right index finger and 70% on the left toe. Both pulse oximeter waveforms are good, and he is warm. His capillary refill time is <3 seconds. His blood pressure reads 75/45 mmHg at the upper limb and 60/30 mmHg at the lower limb. If the lower limb pulse oximetry and blood pressure was to drop further, then the next best management option is:

A. Maintenance fluids of 10% dextrose
B. Starting this patient on an infusion of metariminol
C. Giving a small bolus dose of ephedrine
D. Starting a prostaglandin infusion
E. Starting inhaled nitric oxide

Question 12

An arterial blood gas sample was drawn an hour ago. You decide to analyse it as it was difficult to collect the sample. Choose one statement from below which most accurately describes any errors that might occur.

A. The pH would be raised because of the influx of H+ into cells.
B. The $PaCO_2$ would be unaffected.
C. The haemoglobin concentration would be lower because of haemolysis.
D. The lactate would be increased because of ongoing metabolism.
E. The glucose concentration would increase because of efflux from cells.

Question 13

Examination of the cardiovascular system involves identification of S1, S2 and any associated murmurs. Which one of the following statements regarding the cardiac cycle is true?

A. S1 signifies the closure of the tricuspid and mitral valves only.
B. S1 signifies the end of systole.
C. S2 occurs at the beginning of the T wave.
D. Isovolumetric relaxation occurs during S1.
E. Isovolumetric contraction causes S2.

Question 14

A 50-year-old biomedical researcher was prescribed trimethoprim as prophylaxis after a cystoscopy. Being a scientist himself, he requested more information from the doctor in terms of its action. Choose one statement from the list below which would be most accurate to give to this man regarding trimethoprim:

A. Stimulates purine synthesis.
B. Inhibits the enzyme dihydropterate synthetase.
C. Causes adverse effects that can be lessened by simultaneous administration of folinic acid.
D. Resistance has not been observed in microorganisms.
E. Is less potent than sulfamethoxazole.

Question 15

A 28-week premature baby is delivered in the delivery room. The paediatricians administer prophylactic synthetic surfactant via an endotracheal tube to minimize the incidence of respiratory distress syndrome. Which of the following physical characteristics of the surfactant is responsible for preventing alveolar collapse?

A. It acts as a physical scaffold.
B. It increases surface tension.
C. It generates a variable surface tension.
D. It results in an increase in alveolar pressure.
E. Electrostatic forces hold the alveoli static.

Question 16

You are reviewing the report of an echocardiogram (ECG) of a 72-year-old woman scheduled for a revision of hip replacement. Her ejection fraction is estimated to be 35%. Which one of the following is true?

A. An ejection fraction of 35% roughly equates to 35 mL/beat of blood ejected by the left ventricle.
B. Ejection fraction = (End diastolic volume – End systolic volume)/End systolic volume.
C. Ejection fraction = (End diastolic volume – End systolic volume)/End diastolic volume.
D. Stroke work is calculated by integrating stroke volume against heart rate.
E. Increasing preload does not influence ejection fraction.

Question 17

A medical representative visits the anaesthetic department to provide information to anaesthetists on the drug sugammadex. Which statement is true of sugammadex?

A. Sugammadex displaces muscle relaxants from nicotinic receptors, thereby reversing neuromuscular blockade.
B. The complex of sugammadex and rocuronium binds to plasma proteins.
C. Sugammadex metabolites are found in the urine.
D. The elimination half-life of sugammadex is 18 hours, and the estimated rate of clearance from the plasma is 8.8 mL/min.
E. The recommended dose of sugammadex depends on the level of neuromuscular blockade to be reversed and varies from 2 to 16 mg/kg.

Question 18

Choose the most correct statement regarding temperature measurement in the operating room.

A. Resistance thermometers are not employed as they are not accurate at body temperature.
B. The resistance of thermistors changes linearly with increasing temperature.
C. The junctional potential of a thermocouple increases linearly with increasing temperature.
D. Thermistors are not compatible with wheatstone bridges.
E. The resistance of a platinum wire thermometer decreases exponentially with increasing temperature.

Question 19

A patient who has suffered an acute myocardial infarction is being treated on the intensive therapy unit (ITU) for a low cardiac output state. Which of the following manoeuvers is unlikely to improve his cardiac output?

A. Optimizing preload
B. Increasing afterload
C. Increasing contractility
D. Treating arrhythmias
E. Increasing his diastolic pressure

Question 20

Which of the following patient groups is most suited for primary therapy with hydrochlorothiazide, as an antihypertensive agent?

A. Patients with gout
B. Patients with hyperlipidaemia
C. Young hypertensive patients with rapid resting heart rates
D. African Caribbean patients and elderly patients
E. Patients with impaired renal function

Question 21

A fixed-volume closed system of air at 20°C contains 5 mgm^{-3} of water vapour. Which of the following is true if the system was heated to 23°C?

A. Absolute humidity would decrease.
B. Relative humidity would decrease.
C. Absolute humidity would increase.
D. Relative humidity would increase.
E. Humidity would remain unchanged.

Question 22

You are called to review a 56-year-old woman in the accident and emergency department. She has a background of mild renal impairment secondary to type 2 diabetes. She complains of pleuritic chest pain and is peripherally warm and well perfused with a capillary refill time of 1 second. Her heart rate is 108 beats per minute, blood pressure is 89/65 mmHg despite 2 L of fluid resuscitation and respiratory rate is 28/min with peripheral saturations of 99% on 1 L nasal specs oxygen. Arterial blood gas shows oxygen partial pressure (pO_2) 11 kPa, carbon dioxide partial pressure (pCO_2) 6.8 kPa, pH 7.15, base excess (BE) –8 and lactate 3.8.

Which of the following is she most likely to have?

A. Cardiogenic shock
B. Hypovolaemic shock
C. Septic shock
D. Anaphylactic shock
E. Neurogenic shock

Question 23

The curves in the graph given here demonstrate the various context-sensitive half-lives of drugs. Which of the curves represents remifentanil?

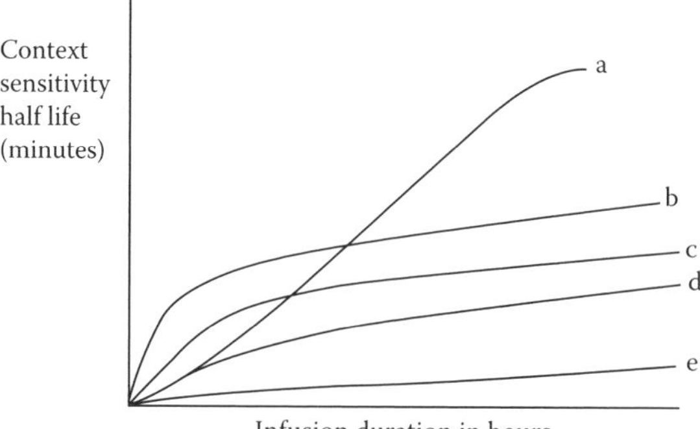

A. a
B. b
C. c
D. d
E. e

Question 24

Which of the following regarding the von Recklinghausen oscillotonometer is correct?

A. It consists of two non-overlapping cuffs.
B. A stethoscope is used to identify the systolic pressure.
C. Maximal oscillations occur at the start of blood flow.
D. The systolic pressure is determined by measuring the occluding cuff.
E. The sensing cuff is larger than the occluding cuff.

Question 25

A 21-year-old man is brought into the accident and emergency department after having been found floating facedown in a lake. Cardiopulmonary resuscitation (CPR) was started by bystanders and is ongoing. His body temperature is currently 30.0°C. Which of the following is most likely to manifest on the ECG?

A. Ventricular fibrillation
B. J-waves
C. Bifid P-waves
D. Tall tented T-waves
E. T-wave inversion inferiorly

Question 26

You consent a patient for a phase II (clinical-testing) trial of a new drug. The patient would like to know the research process for any drug development. In which order does the drug development process occur?

A. *In vitro* studies > animal testing > clinical testing (phases I, II and III) > marketing (phase IV)
B. Animal studies > *in vitro* studies > clinical testing (phases I, II and III) > marketing (phase IV)
C. Animal studies > clinical testing (phases I, II and III) > marketing (phase IV) > *in vitro* studies
D. *In vitro* studies > animal testing > marketing > clinical testing
E. *In vitro* studies > clinical testing > animal studies > marketing

Question 27

During a prolonged craniotomy for tumour resection, an infusion of vecuronium was used to prevent movement. At the end of the procedure, double burst stimulation (DBS) was used to assess residual neuromuscular blockade. Which of the following statements regarding DBS is most correct?

A. Fade is elicited even if suxamethonium has been used.
B. DBS is more sensitive than train of four.
C. Each burst contains two impulses at supramaximal current.
D. The negative electrode should be placed proximally.
E. Each burst is separated by 500 ms.

Question 28

A very anxious 25-year-old woman is listed for a hysteroscopy. She tells you she suffers from palpitations 1–2 times a week which are associated with panic attacks. She is a smoker and has been nil by mouth for 12 hours. A 12-lead ECG performed that morning shows a sinus tachycardia with a rate of 118. Which one of the following is most unlikely to be the cause of her tachycardia?

A. Increased B1 activation due to anxiety
B. Hypovolaemia
C. Nicotine
D. Wolfe–Parkinson–White syndrome
E. Activation of M2 receptors

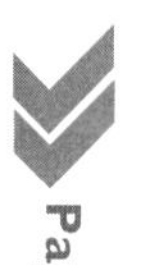

Question 29

A previously fit 65-year-old man has undergone a prolonged (2 hours) transurethral resection of the prostrate (TURP) under general anaesthesia. He is transferred to the recovery area with a laryngeal mask airway (LMA) *in situ.* Forty-five minutes later, you are called by the recovery nurse as the patient has not regained consciousness. His cardiorespiratory parameters are stable. Which of the following options is most likely to cause this clinical scenario?

A. Cerebrovascular accident
B. Hypercarbia
C. Residual anaesthetic effect
D. Hyponatremia
E. Hypoglycaemia

Question 30

Regarding the ECG, which of the following statements is true?

A. The electric potential at the electrode is 90 mvolts.
B. The bandwidth is usually 0.5–80 Hz.
C. The signal is composed of superimposed square waves.
D. CM5 configuration is normally adopted to assess arrhythmias.
E. Signal amplification is avoided, as it causes signal degradation.

PAPER 2 ANSWERS

Answer 1: D

The Bain circuit is a coaxial Mapleson D breathing system and has a low resistance to gas flow. Fresh gas flow (FGF) is delivered by the smaller inner tube housed within the larger corrugated tubing. During inspiration, gas housed in the corrugated tubing and FGF from the inner tubing are breathed in. During expiration, gas is expelled into the outer tubing and mixes with the FGF from the inner tubing. Some of this is vented via the adjustable pressure-limiting (APL) valve situated distally. During the expiratory pause, FGF replaces the expired gas within larger corrugated tubing which is vented by the adjustable APL. The APL valve can incorporate a scavenging system. This arrangement is not efficient for spontaneous breathing, and flow rates of 200–300 mL/kg are required. During positive pressure ventilation, however, the system becomes efficient, and FGF of 70 mL/kg is enough to achieve normocarbia.

Further reading

Anaesthesia UK. Mapleson D. http://www.frca.co.uk/article.aspx?articleid=100141

Answer 2: B

An approximate dose regimen for a 70 kg patient would be:

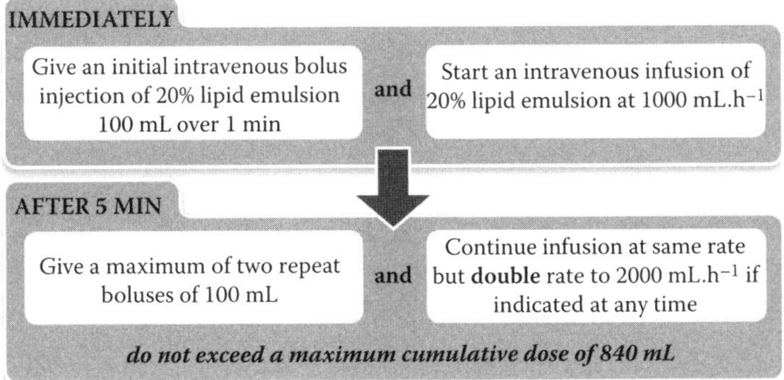

Further reading

Cave, G., Harrop-Griffiths, W. (Chair), Harvey, M., Meek, T., Picard, J., Short, T., and Weinberg, G. AAGBI safety guideline. http://www.aagbi.org/sites/default/files/la_toxicity_notes_2010_0.pdf (From the Association of Anaesthetists Great Britain and Ireland (AAG-BI), London.)

Answer 3: A

Action potentials are all-or-nothing events. Stimuli come in various intensities, and once the stimulus intensity reaches a particular threshold level, only then is an action potential elicited. Whether a stimulus is of the threshold intensity or above it, it will trigger an action potential. The size of the stimulus therefore matters, and when the intensity of the stimulus is below threshold an action potential is not generated.

An action potential is propagated along the neuronal axon–cell surface through the sequential depolarization and repolarization of the cell membrane. The process is sped up by the presence of a myelin sheath. Interruptions in the myelin sheath along the axon are called the *nodes of Ranvier* and contain a high density of ion channels involved in axon potential propagation. The myelin is an insulator and so the action potential 'jumps' from node to node – this is termed *saltatory transmission* whereby depolarization in one node of Ranvier induces depolarization in the adjacent node. This method of nerve conduction is faster than if the myelin sheath were not present and adjacent areas of cell membrane were being depolarized.

Action potentials involve positive feedback mechanisms – see the reference here.

Further reading

Power, I., and Kam, P. *Principles of Physiology for the Anaesthetist*. 2nd ed. London: Hodder Arnold, 2008, 7–16.

Answer 4: B

The Severinghaus electrode is a modified pH electrode that is used to measure the CO_2 tension. The apparatus houses a hydrogen-sensitive glass probe, encased in a nylon mesh that is impregnated with a bicarbonate solution. Two electrodes are placed on either side of the probe, one on the inside of the glass electrode and one in the buffer. A plastic membrane permeable to CO_2 separates the sample from the system. CO_2 from the sample diffuses across this semipermeable membrane and reacts with bicarbonate and water within the mesh, resulting in a change in the pH. This change is measured by the electrode and relates directly to the carbon dioxide tension. If the membrane is damaged, then other molecules are able to enter and react with the bicarbonate, which renders the system inaccurate for CO_2 measurement. The response time (2–3 minutes) is slower than a pH electrode as the CO_2 has to diffuse across the membrane. The system is maintained at 37°C.

Further reading

Davies. P., and Kenny, G. *Basic Physics and Measurement in Anaesthesia*. 5th ed. London: Butterworth Heinemann, 2005.

Answer 5: C

Ketorolac has a half-life of 6 hours. It is a non-steroidal anti-inflammatory drug (NSAID). It is used for its analgesic, anti-inflamatory and antipyretic actions. It is a cyclooxygenase inhibitor, thus preventing the formation of prostaglandins. The drug can be given intramuscularly (IM). The IM available dosings are 15, 30 and 60 mg. 10 mg of ketorolac has the analgesic equivalence of either 50 mg pethidine or 6 mg morphine. However, ketorolac causes less drowsiness, nausea and vomiting than opioids. In some patients, ketorolac should be used with caution as it inhibits platelet aggregation and may prolong bleeding time. Some of its contraindications are bronchospasm, angioedema and avoidance in patients with nasal polyps.

Further reading

Peck, T.E., Williams, M., and Hill, S.A. *Pharmacology for Anaesthesia and Intensive Care*. Cambridge: Cambridge University Press, 2003.

Answer 6: C

The vomiting centre located in the medulla receives afferents from multiple sources. The cerebral cortex (pain and anxiety), chemoreceptors and baroreceptors from the gut, pain receptors from the periphery, and organ of balance (cerebellum, labyrinths and vestibular apparatus – cholinergic) all supply afferents into the vomiting centre. The chemoreceptor trigger zone is a collection of cells located outside of the blood–brain barrier in the floor of the fourth ventricle. Raised intracranial pressure is thought to cause a direct pressure effect on these cells causing nausea. It is thought that dopamine and 5HT3 receptors play a role in the stimulation of these cells. Chemotherapeutic agents and other emetogenic drugs are thought to exert such an effect at this zone. The chemoreceptor trigger zone stimulates the vomiting centre in turn.

Answer 7: A

A small amount (100–300 microlitres, or μL) of sample is usually passed through four electrodes. The system is maintained at a constant temperature of 37°C and incorporates a Clarke electrode (arterial blood gas, or PaO_2), a Severinghaus electrode (arterial carbon dioxide tension, or $PaCO_2$), a pH electrode and a fourth reference electrode. Often, the analysers also directly measure haemoglobin concentration and ion concentrations (e.g. sodium, potassium, calcium and lactate). Derived values are generated from this data and include the bicarbonate concentration, base excess and oxygen content and saturation.

Further reading

Davey, A., and Diba, A. *Ward's Anaesthetic Equipment*. 5th ed. London: Elsevier Saunders, 2005.

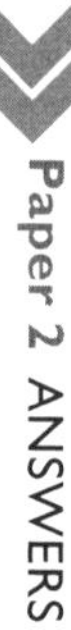

Answer 8: E

This is a case of a primary psychotic disorder, schizophrenia. The drug of choice for this patient is resperidone. Resperidone is an atypical antipsychotic that would treat this patient's auditory hallucinations and paranoid delusions.

Benztropine has no antipsychotic properties that would benefit this patient. It is an anticholinergic that is used with haloperidol (a typical antipsychotic) to control extrapyramidal symptoms.

Diazepam is a long-acting benzodiazepine. It is used in the management of an anxiety disorder. Lorazepam, a shorter-acting benzodiazepine, is used adjunctively in psychotic individuals for acute agitation.

Fluoxetine is a selective serotonin reuptake inhibitor (SSRI) used in depression.

Lithium is used in bipolar disorder. Although individuals with bipolar disorder may have delusions, they are usually of a grandiose quality.

In such individuals, antipsychotic medications like risperidone can be given as well because lithium takes approximately 10 days to have a beneficial effect. However, this patient has profound paranoid delusions suggestive of schizophrenia.

Answer 9: B

The stomach contributes to the mechanical and biochemical digestion of food and contains a variety of highly specialized cells which produce and regulate the production of acid, digestive enzymes and mucus. Fundal parietal cells produce HCl at a concentration of 0.15 M which helps protein breakdown, activates pepsinogen, augments absorption of iron and calcium and kills ingested pathogens. Chief cells produce pepsin which is a proteolytic enzyme. Intrinsic factor is produced by parietal cells and is essential in the absorption of B_{12}. Intrinsic factor combines with B_{12} to form a complex which is protected from destruction by enzymes, and is absorbed in the terminal ileum. Mucus forms a protective mechanical layer on the surface of the stomach, protecting it from the strongly acidic conditions and proteolytic enzymes.

Further reading

Jolliffe, D.M. Practical gastric physiology. *Contin Educ Anaesth Crit Care Pain* (2009) 9 (6): 173–7.

Answer 10: E

Cardiac muscle is a specialized form of muscle cell. It contains actin and myosin, with troponin and tropomyosin arranged as in striated muscle, but the muscle cells are branched and are connected to each other via desmosomes and gap junctions to form a functional syncitium. This allows the action potential to travel from cell to cell, thus allowing a wave of coordinated muscle contraction. When an action potential reaches a cardiomyocyte, it induces the opening of voltage-gated ion channels. This results in a rapid depolarization of the myocyte (phase 0).

These time-dependent sodium channels are rapidly inactivated, and there is a small leakage of K out of the cell, causing a partial repolarization. This K efflux is balanced by an influx of Ca via L-type Ca channels which causes the plateau phase. The calcium influx during this phase causes 'calcium-induced calcium release' from the sarcoplasmic reticulum and causes an almost exponential increase in the intracellular calcium concentration. This augments actin–myosin cross-bridge formation and muscle contraction. The Na–Ca exchanger prolongs the late stages of the plateau current, and myocyte repolarization is mediated by slow-activating voltage-gated K channels.

Further reading

Levick, J.R. *An Introduction to Cardiovascular Physiology*. 4th ed. London: Hodder Arnold, 2003, 24–43.

Answer 11: D

This baby has a congenital cardiac disease of coarctation of the aorta that presents with differential blood pressures and pulse oximetry in the upper and lower limbs. The perfusion of the lower limb would still rely on the ductus arteriosus (newborn), and thus prostaglandins would help keep the ductus arteriosus patent and perfuse the trunk and lower extremities. Prostaglandin is known to cause respiratory and circulatory depression, thus monitoring of the airway and blood pressure care are crucial during therapy.

Although 10% dextrose may help the developing brain if blood sugars are low, it would not reverse the clinical parameters in the question.

Metariminol infusions are not used in babies. Ephedrine again would not be beneficial in maintaining an open duct. Inhaled nitric oxide is useful as a therapy for pulmonary hypertension, However, in this situation, pulmonary vasodilation would reverse the duct flow and worsen the hypotension in the lower limb.

Further reading

Peck, T.E., Williams, M., and Hill, S.A. *Pharmacology for Anaesthesia and Intensive Care*. Cambridge: Cambridge University Press, 2003.

Answer 12: D

Errors in blood gas analysis frequently occur as a consequence of incorrect handling of samples. Prolonged storage at room temperature results in ongoing cellular metabolism and in a lower pH, PaO_2 and glucose concentration. The $PaCO_2$ would increase during aerobic metabolism, and lactate would increase in anaerobic metabolism. During prolonged storage, cooling is advised to reduce errors. However, rapid cooling may result in haemolysis which would increase the potassium concentration.

Air bubbles in the sample must be expelled immediately, as the presence would result in a lower $PaCO_2$ and higher PaO_2.

Clots might occur if the sample is not mixed immediately or if heparin is not used, and this would result in an increased potassium concentration. Furthermore, dilution of the sample with excess heparin would result in a lower $PaCO_2$, base excess and bicarbonate, mimicking a metabolic acidosis. Additionally, as heparin is anionic, it also adsorbs positively charged ions and may result in falsely low readings.

Further reading

Radiometer Medical ApS. Avoiding preanalytical errors – in blood gas testing. 2008. http://www.radiometer.com/en/services/~/media/Files/RadiometerComCloneset/Parent/en/Miscellaneous%20Items/990-550_201104D%20Avoiding%20Handbook%20en_low.pdf

Sood, P., Paul, G., and Puri, S. Interpretation of arterial blood gas. *Ind J C Care Med* (2010) 14 (2): 57–64.

Answer 13: A

The first heart sound signifies the closure of the mitral and tricuspid valves at the beginning of systole, during which the pulmonary and aortic valves open. The second heart sound signifies the closure of the pulmonary and aortic valves at the beginning of diastole, during which time the mitral and tricuspid valves open. Systole coincides with the electrocardiogram (ECG) from the beginning QRS complex until the T-wave has become iso-electric. Diastole coincides with the ECG from this point until the beginning of the next QRS complex. The cardiac cycle can be divided into five phases:

Phase 1: atrial contraction (during diastole);

Phase 2: ventricular iso-volumetric contraction and onset of systole – causing closure of mitral and tricuspid valves (S1). The aortic and pulmonary valves are still closed at this point until a sufficient pressure is generated in the ventricles to cause these valves to open; leading to

Phase 3: ventricular ejection – during the end of which the pressure gradient across the aortic and pulmonary valves is reversed; leading to

Phase 4: closure of aortic and pulmonary valves (S2) and iso-volumetric relaxation of the ventricle (beginning of diastole); and

Phase 5: opening of the mitral and tricuspid valves and ventricular filling by passive flow from the atria.

Further reading

Cross, M., and Plunkett, E. *Physics, Pharmacology and Physiology for Anaesthetists.* Cambridge: Cambridge University Press, 2008, 146–8.

Yentis, S., Hirsch, N., and Smith, G. *Anaesthesia and Intensive Care A–Z.* 4th ed. London: Churchill Livingstone, 2009.

Answer 14: C

Trimethoprim inhibits the production of purines and pyrimidine bases by inhibition of the enzyme dihydrofolate reductase. Its adverse effects can be lessened by simultaneous administration of folinic acid. Some Gram-negative bacteria have been observed to rely on an altered dihydrofolate reductase enzyme, thus proving resistant to trimethoprim. Trimethoprim is more potent than sulfamethoxazole.

Further reading

Peck, T.E., Williams, M., and Hill, S.A. *Pharmacology for Anaesthesia and Intensive Care*. Cambridge: Cambridge University Press, 2003.

Answer 15: C

Surfactants produced by type II pneumocytes are complex molecules containing phospholipids and apoproteins. They prevent alveolar collapse by variably changing the surface tension. La Place's law states that the pressure gradient across the wall of a sphere with a gas–liquid interface is determined by 2× the tension or radius. In the alveoli the water on the inner surface has a surface tension which will tend to collapse the structure, and smaller alveoli would be expected to empty into larger ones. Such collapse *in vivo* is prevented by the incorporation of surfactant. These molecules are repulsive to each other and hence reduce the tension. As the alveoli empty, the concentration of surfactant increases, thereby reducing surface tension. At higher volumes, there is less reduction of surface tension. This differential prevents the emptying of smaller alveoli into larger alveoli.

Further reading

Davies, P., and Kenny, G. *Basic Physics and Measurement in Anaesthesia*. 5th ed. London: Butterworth Heinemann, 2005.

Answer 16: C

Ejection fraction refers to the fraction of the end diastolic volume of the left ventricle which is ejected during systole. The fraction can be multiplied by 100 to give a percentage. The stroke work of the left ventricle refers to the work done by the myocardium with each contraction. It can be calculated from the area contained within a pressure-versus-volume loop.

As the pre-load is increased, the volume component of the equation increases and thus the stroke work increases.

Increasing afterload increases the pressure component, and thus stroke work is increased too.

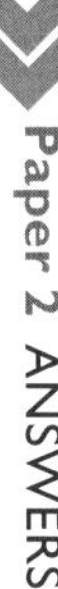

Further reading

Cross, M., and Plunkett, E. *Physics, Pharmacology and Physiology for Anaesthetists.* Cambridge: Cambridge University Press, 2008, 155–6, 162–6.

Answer 17: E

Sugammadex binds to neuromuscular blocking agents like rocuronium and vecuronium to form complexes. Formation of these complexes removes drug from the neuromuscular junction, thus reversing neuromuscular blockade. Both sugammadex and rocuronium will bind to plasma proteins.

In preclinical and clinical studies, renal excretion of the unchanged product of sugammadex has been observed with no metabolites being formed.

The elimination half-life of sugammadex is 1.8 hours, the plasma clearance is 88 mL/min and greater than 90% is excreted in the first 24 hours following administration. The therapeutic dose of sugammadex depends on the degree of neuromuscular blockade to be reversed and varies from 2 to 16 mg.

Further reading

Anaesthesia UK. Neuromuscular blockade and reversal. http://www.frca.co.uk/sectioncontents.aspx?sectionid=84

Answer 18: C

Temperature can be measured using electrical techniques which incorporate the resistance wire thermometer, thermistors and thermocouples. Resistance wire thermometers incorporate a length of platinum and are very accurate in the range of 0–100°C. However, they have a relatively slow response time. In this system, the resistance of the wire increases linearly with increasing temperature. Thermistors are composed of metal oxides and respond rapidly to small changes in temperature. Rising temperature causes an exponential fall in resistance. Thermocouples contain two different metals which give rise to a potential difference (the Seebeck effect). This potential difference is dependent on temperature such that as temperature increases, there is a proportional increase in the potential difference. The sensitivity of all electrical methods of temperature measurement is increased if the probes are incorporated into a wheatstone bridge.

Further reading

Anaesthesia UK. Temperature measurement: electrical techniques. 2005. http://www.frca.co.uk/article.aspx?articleid=100326

Davies. P., and Kenny, G. *Basic Physics and Measurement in Anaesthesia.* 5th ed. London: Butterworth Heinemann, 2005.

Answer 19: B

Cardiac output is the product of stroke volume and heart rate. Tachycardia increases cardiac output at the expense of increasing myocardial work and oxygen consumption. Bradycardia allows for a greater diastolic filling time and myocardial perfusion time, but at extremes of bradycardia, this advantage is overridden and cardiac output decreases. Stroke volume depends on preload, afterload and contractility. The effect of preload on stroke volume and cardiac output is demonstrated by Frank Starling's famous curve.

As a muscle fibre is stretched (i.e. preload is increased), the force of the muscle contraction (i.e. stroke volume) increases up to a point, after which it plateaus.

Contractility (force of contraction at a given muscle length) can be increased and can also increase stroke volume.

Afterload (analogous to systemic vascular resistance [SVR]) is an essential component of the blood pressure and organ perfusion pressure. Increases in the afterload tend to decrease cardiac output as the ventricle has a resistance against which to eject.

Any rhythm which disrupts the synchronized contraction of cardiac muscle is also likely to decrease cardiac output. Furthermore, the lack of atrial contraction can lead to a lower ejected volume, as the 'atrial kick' contributes to ventricular end diastolic volume.

Increasing diastolic pressure augments cardiac muscle perfusion and is likely to help an ischaemic myocardium.

Further reading

Levick, J.R. *An Introduction to Cardiovascular Physiology*. 4th ed. London: Hodder Arnold, 2003, 70–95.

Answer 20: D

African Caribbean and elderly patients are better treated with diuretics than with beta blockers or angiotensin-converting enzyme (ACE) inhibitors. The hyperuricemia caused by thiazides can precipitate an attack in patients with gout. Another adverse effect of thiazides is low-density lipoprotein (LDL) cholesterolemia that can increase the risk of complications in hyperlipidemic patients. A young hypertensive patient with a rapid resting heart rate will benefit from beta blockade. Unlike furosemide, thiazides are not a good option in patients with impaired renal function as they are not able to increase sodium output in a failing kidney.

Further reading

Peck, T.E., Williams, M., and Hill, S.A. *Pharmacology for Anaesthesia and Intensive Care*. Cambridge: Cambridge University Press, 2003.

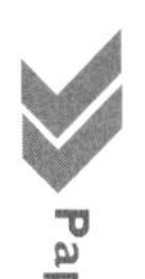

Answer 21: B

Absolute humidity (AH) is the total mass of water in a given volume of gas. As the temperature of an open system (where water vapour can be added) increases, AH would increase. In the above example, however, AH would not change. Relative humidity is determined by the following equation:

Relative humidity = AH / mass of water required to fully saturate the system

Relative humidity is often expressed as a percentage.

In the closed system described here, no further water can be added and hence the relative humidity would decrease (as temperature rises, the amount of water required to saturate would increase).

Further reading

Anaesthesia UK. Humidity. 2010. http://www.frca.co.uk/article.aspx?articleid=239

Wilkes, A.R. Humidification: its importance and delivery. *Contin Educ Anaesth Crit Care Pain* (2001) 1(2): 40–3.

Answer 22: C

It is likely that this woman is in septic shock as she is peripherally warm and hyperdynamic. There is evidence of inadequate organ perfusion as exhibited by the metabolic acidosis, and pneumonia is likely to be the root cause. There is no history suggestive of trauma; however, a rare epidural abscess causing neurogenic shock cannot be excluded. Hypovolaemic and cardiogenic shock usually manifest with the patient being cool and peripherally shut down.

Further reading

Yentis, S., Hirsch, N., and Smith, G. *Anaesthesia and Intensive Care A–Z.* 4th ed. London: Churchill Livingstone, 2009.

Answer 23: E

The half-life of agents given as a continuous infusion is dependent on the duration of infusion. This is known as the context-sensitive half-life. The graph below demonstrates the context-sensitive half-lives of common anaesthetic agents that are often infused in clinical practice (a = fentanyl, b = thiopentone, c = midazolam, d = alfentanil, e = remifentanil).

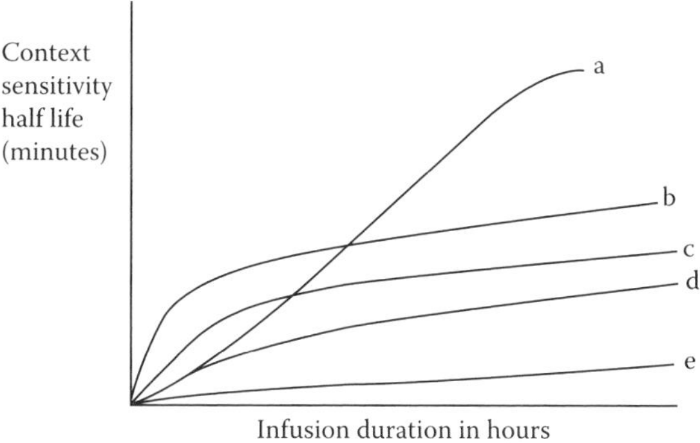

Answer 24: D

The von Recklinghausen oscillotonometer consists of two overlapping cuffs (a large occluding one and a smaller sensing one), a valve which allows deflation of the cuffs and a needle gauge to measure pressure within the cuffs. A lever is also incorporated which allows for switching the needle gauge between the cuffs. This arrangement allows blood pressure (BP) measurement without a stethoscope. The cuffs are inflated to above systolic pressure, and the needle gauge is set to measure the pressure in the sensing cuff which amplifies the signal. The pressure is then slowly released via the valve. As the systolic pressure is reached, the needle begins to oscillate. Deflation is stopped at this point, and the lever is turned to measure the pressure in the occluding cuff. At mean arterial pressure, the maximal oscillations are seen, and at diastolic pressure oscillations begin to vanish. Measurement at these points will allow determination of the relevant pressures.

Further reading

Ward, M., and Langton, J.A. Blood pressure measurement. *Contin Educ Anaesth Crit Care Pain* (2007) 7 (4): 122–6.

Answer 25: B

The ECG is a recording of the electrical activity of the heart taken from various angles and from between sets of leads. The electrical activity of the heart changes with insults to the heart, and thus the ECG can be diagnostic of various pathologies. With hypothermia, J-waves and ventricular arrhythmias are seen at 30°C, with ventricular fibrillation (VF) usually occurring at 28°C. J-waves are benign and carry no clinical significance. Bifid P-waves occur with atrial enlargement. Tall tented T-waves are seen with hyperkalaemia, and T-wave inversion is usually seen in ischaemic cardiac states.

Further reading

Yentis, S., Hirsch, N., and Smith, G. *Anaesthesia and Intensive Care A–Z*. 4th ed. London: Churchill Livingstone, 2009.

Answer 26: A

The discovery of a drug, its development and its final approval for patient use can take 10 to 15 years on an average. The approval process of a drug before it is approved for human use is as follows:

1. *In vitro* studies and animal studies ascertain the safety of the drug formulation and its action.
2. Phase I trials determine safety and dosage in a small group (100) of volunteers.
3. Phase II is to assess the drug's effectiveness and detect adverse effects in a larger group (typically 500 volunteers).
4. Phase III is to confirm its effectiveness and monitor its side effects in a much bigger group (5000 volunteers) over a longer duration.
5. The drug and approval process is reviewed by the U.S. Food and Drug Administration (FDA) and the Medicines and Healthcare Products Regulatory Agency (MHRA).
6. Phase IV is additional post-marketing testing.

Further reading

PhRMA. http://www.phrma.org

Answer 27: B

In double burst stimulation (DBS), two bursts of supramaximal current at 50 Hz are applied 750 ms apart. Each burst contains three impulses that have a duration of 0.2 ms each and are separated by 20 ms. The supramaximal current applied at the skin is usually in 50–60 mAmps and is defined as a current 25% higher than that required to stimulate all nerve fibres. In unparalysed muscle, two twitches of equal strength will occur. When residual neuromuscular blockade is present, the twitch height of the second burst is smaller than the first and a DBS ratio can be generated. This ratio has similar properties to the train of four (TOF) ratio. Tactile evaluation of the DBS signal is more accurate than the TOF. As with the TOF, fade is absent in DBS, when suxamethonium is used. Instead, both twitch heights are reduced. In the TOF test, a supramaximal current is applied at 2 Hz (i.e. 4 impulses, 0.5 seconds apart).

Further reading

Conor, D., McGrath, C., and Hunter, J.M. Monitoring of neuromuscular block. *Contin Educ Anaesth Crit Care Pain* (2006) 6 (1): 7–12.

Answer 28: E

The cardiac impulse is generated in the pacemaker cells of the heart – the sino-atrial node. This rate of firing of the cells can be modified by several factors. The node is primarily under the control of the autonomic nervous system. Parasympathetic fibres release acetylcholine which acts on muscarinc type-2 receptors, resulting in the hyperpolarization of the pacemaker cells and thus increasing the duration taken for the cells to reach the threshold potential. The reverse is true for sympathetic stimulation mediated by B_1 receptors, commonly in response to anxiety, hypovolamia and pain. Sympathetic stimulation tends to lower the threshold potential and hence increases the rate at which threshold levels for firing of action potentials are reached.

Nicotine and caffeine are both stimulants. Nicotine stimulates the ACH receptors on the adrenal medulla, causing release of adrenaline and noradrenaline. Caffeine inhibits the breakdown of cyclic adenosine monophosphate (cAMP) and thus augments B adrenoceptor activity.

Further reading

Levick, J.R. *An Introduction to Cardiovascular Physiology*. 4th ed. London: Hodder Arnold, 2003, 44–57.

News Medical. Caffeine pharmacology. http://www.news-medical.net/health/Caffeine-Pharmacology.aspx

Answer 29: D

The most likely diagnosis here is transurethral resection of the prostrate (TURP) syndrome that has resulted from prolonged duration of surgery causing hyponatremia and unconsciousness. TURP syndrome can go unrecognized in patients given a general anaesthetic as the central nervous system (CNS) signs are masked. Excessive absorption of irrigant fluid into the circulation leads to increased intravascular volume, and hyponatremia and low serum osmolality ensue. Systemically, it causes the following:

- Cardiovascular system (CVS): bradycardia, hypotension, hypertension and ECG changes due to hyponatremia (wide QRS, ST elevations, and ventricular tachycardia [VT] and ventricular fibrillation [VF] arrhythmia);
- Respiratory: pulmonary oedema secondary to fluid overload; and
- CNS: confusion, coma, seizures and visual disturbances.
- Some factors which increase the incidence of TURP syndrome are as follows:
  - Prolonged duration of surgery (>60 minutes);
  - Haemorrhage leading to absorption of irrigant fluid from the open prostatic sinuses; and
  - Increased height of irrigant fluid, thus increasing hydrostatic pressure and greater absorption of irrigant fluid.

The management for this patient would be to treat his hyponatremia with hypertonic saline (3%) or haemofiltration. Diuretics should be reserved for patients with fluid overload. He should be managed on the high-dependency unit (HDU) with invasive lines (arterial or central venous pressure [CVP]) if needed. Hypercarbia, residual anaesthetic effect and hypoglycemia are unlikely causes here.

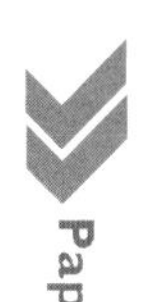

Further reading

Peck, T.E., Williams, M., and Hill, S.A. *Pharmacology for Anaesthesia and Intensive Care*. Cambridge: Cambridge University Press, 2003.

Answer 30: B

The ECG measures the electric potential of the myocardium at the skin. In the myocardium, the potential is as high as 90 mvolts, but at the skin it is reduced to only 1–2 mvolts and hence amplification of the signal is vital. The ECG signal is a complex arrangement of superimposed sine waves. The fundamental frequency is the slowest of these. In order for the amplified signal to represent the original signal, a sufficient range of frequencies needs to be amplified (bandwidth). The bandwidth must include the fundamental frequency and usually eight further harmonics. Typically the bandwidth is 0.5–80 Hz. A lower bandwidth will result in artefacts from breathing, while a higher range will result in interference arising from muscle twitches and nearby electric equipment. The CM5 configuration is useful for detecting left ventricular ischaemia and involves placing the right arm electrode on the manubrium and the left arm electrode at the V5 position. The remaining electrode can be placed anywhere else but is often placed on the left shoulder. Lead I should be analyzed.

Further reading

Brown, Z., and Gupta, B. Biological signals and their measurement update in anaesthesia. 2008. http://update.anaesthesiologists.org/2008/12/01/biological-signals-and-their-measurement/

Lee, J. ECG monitoring in theatre. *Update Anaesthes* (2000) (11): Article 5.

5 PAPER 3 QUESTIONS

Question 1

Which of the following statements regarding electricity is correct?

A. One volt is defined as the potential difference across a wire carrying 1 amp of current.
B. One ampere can be defined as the flow of one coulomb of electrons past one point in one minute.
C. A thinner metal wire has higher resistance than a thicker one.
D. Resistance can be defined as the potential difference times the current.
E. Power is expressed in joules.

Question 2

A 55-year-old man is scheduled for an oesophagectomy and undergoes peri-operative cardiopulmonary exercise testing. Which of the following cardiac changes would you not see during his test?

A. Tachycardia
B. Decrease of vagal tone
C. Isolated rise in systolic blood pressure (BP)
D. Increased sympathetic tone
E. Increased venous return

Question 3

Anaesthetic trainees attend a pharmacology refresher course before their Royal College of Anaesthetists (RCOA) single best answer (SBA) exams. The lecture is on isomerism. Which of the following drugs is a tautomer?

A. Mivacurium
B. S-ketamine
C. Midazolam
D. Ibuprofen
E. Racemic bupivacaine

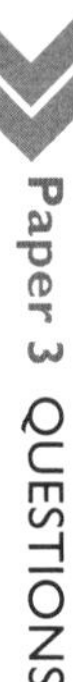

Question 4

Which of the following regarding hot wire anemometry is true?

A. The resistance of the wire drops with cooling.
B. It directly measures gas volumes.
C. It is very sensitive and has a very fast response time.
D. Calibration is not required.
E. It can be used with gas mixtures containing ethyl ether, isoflurane or desflurane.

Question 5

Vascular endothelial dysfunction is implicated in the pathophysiology of multiple diseases. Which of the following is not a function of vascular endothelial cells?

A. Anticoagulation and thrombosis
B. Regulation of vascular tone
C. Preventing the passage of leucocytes during the inflammatory response
D. Angiogenesis
E. Regulating blood tissue exchange

Question 6

A term pregnant woman has undergone an emergency caesarean section for foetal distress. The anaesthetic consisted of an epidural top-up with 20 mL of plain 0.5% bupivacaine and 50 μg fentanyl. Post-delivery, the baby required resuscitation for bupivacaine toxicity. The mechanism for toxicity in this case is due to:

A. Reduced interval between epidural drug bolus and baby delivery
B. Low kPa of bupivacaine in the mother
C. Reduced foetal clearance
D. Ion trapping within foetus
E. Inherited enzyme deficiency

Question 7

Which of the following statements regarding diffusion of a gas across the alveolar membrane is true?

A. It is independent of temperature.
B. It is inversely proportional to the square of the molecular weight.
C. It is proportional to the solubility.
D. It is inversely proportional to the surface area.
E. Oxygen diffuses faster than carbon dioxide.

Question 8

A 70-year-old man is scheduled to have a knee replacement. A peri-operative echocardiography (ECHO) shows elevated pulmonary arterial pressures. Which of the following is likely to exacerbate his pulmonary hypertension?

A. Low PaO_2
B. High PaO_2
C. Low PCO_2
D. Nitric oxide
E. Volatile anaesthetic agents

Question 9

A 50-year-old male is being treated for acute traumatic brain injury on the neurocritical care unit. On the ward round, the nurse mentions that the urine output is adequate but green coloured. The patient is ventilated with remifentanil, propofol and noradrenaline infusions as part of his care. The neurosurgeon had inserted an external ventricular drain (EVD) under local anaesthesia (lignocaine) an hour ago. The green colour of urine is due to which of the following chemical groups?

A. Monoethylglycinexylide metabolite of lignocaine
B. Quinol metabolite of propofol
C. An ester of remifentanil
D. Catechol-O-methyltransferase (COMT) of noradrenaline
E. Methylated noradrenaline

Question 10

A previously fit and well 26-year-old male was involved in a road traffic accident after consuming a large quantity of alcohol. Catastrophic abdominal bleeding is suspected, resuscitation attempts have failed to establish haemodynamic stability and surgical control is the only remaining option. You have induced anaesthesia with 450 mg of thiopentone and suxamethonium. At laryngoscopy, you are unable to intubate despite repositioning the patient. What is the next best course of action?

A. Awaken the patient and re-anaesthetize with senior assistance.
B. Secure the airway with a fibre-optic scope.
C. Needle cricothyroidectomy.
D. Insert a Proseal™ laryngeal mask airway (LMA) and proceed if ventilation is possible.
E. Surgical tracheostomy.

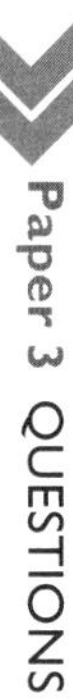

Question 11

A student utilizes Fowler's method to measure the volume of the conducting airways that does not take part in gaseous exchange. Which of the following best describes what the student has measured?

A. Dead space
B. Physiological dead space
C. Alveolar dead space
D. Anatomical dead space
E. Bronchial dead space

Question 12

A 65-year-old male undergoing inguinal hernia surgery under general anaesthesia has a sinus rhythm with a rate of 45/min. His BP is 70/40mm Hg despite fluid challenges. His BP initially increased to 120/80 mm Hg with boluses of ephedrine, but subsequently the BP fell and repeated doses of ephedrine were ineffective. This phenomenon is best explained by the mechanism of:

A. Desensitization
B. Tolerance
C. Tachyphylaxis
D. Allosteric modulation
E. Antagonism

Question 13

Which of the following statements regarding medical magnetic resonance imaging (MRI) scanners is true?

A. They have magnetic field strengths in excess of 30 000 times that of the Earth's field.
B. The Faraday cage contains the generated magnetic field.
C. Superconductors are immersed in liquid hydrogen close to absolute zero.
D. Atoms with paired electrons, such as hydrogen, align with the magnetic field.
E. Gamma rays are used to perturb the magnetic field during image acquisition.

Question 14

Which two variables would allow you to obtain the best estimate of the oxygen content of a sample of blood?

A. Haemoglobin concentration and O_2 saturations
B. Haemoglobin concentration and PaO_2
C. PaO_2 and O_2 saturations
D. PaO_2 and Huffner constant
E. Huffner constant and O_2 saturations

Question 15

The membrane-bound G protein is a group of heterotrimeric proteins. It has a serpentine structure with seven helices that traverse the membrane. Which of the following is also true of G proteins?

A. They prevent a stimulus across the cell membrane.
B. They produce intracellular signal amplification.
C. They are called G proteins because they are linked to glucose.
D. In the active form, the alpha subunit is bound to guanine diphosphate (GDP).
E. Ligand-receptor complex interaction produces alpha-GDP-beta gamma.

Question 16

An intubated 34-year-old female patient is scheduled for an MRI of the brain following a collapse. On arriving to the intensive care unit (ICU), you are advised that the patient is in the second trimester of pregnancy. Furthermore, she had a mitral valve replacement following endocarditis 3 years ago. The porter who is to assist with the transfer is known to have a cardiac pacemaker. Which of the following statements regarding safety during the MRI is most correct?

A. Cardiac pacemakers will not malfunction if kept outside the 50 Gauss line.
B. A patient with sternal wires post valve replacement cannot undergo MRI.
C. Pregnancy is a contraindication for MRI.
D. Ear protection is not necessary in the anaesthetized patient.
E. Oxygen sensors must be installed in the scanning room.

Question 17

A 35-year-old man with acute disseminated intravascular coagulation (DIC) is found to have a thrombus in his portal vein. A portal circulation is best described as follows:

A. A network connecting a venous-to-arterial circulation
B. A network of vessels connecting an arterial-to-venous circulation
C. A network carrying venous blood to a capillary network
D. A network of blood vessels connecting two capillary networks
E. The circulation carrying venous blood from the gut to the liver

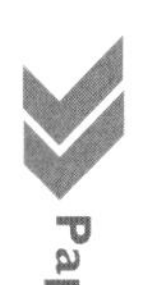

Question 18

Intravenous anaesthetics have been defined as agents that will induce loss of consciousness in one arm-brain circulation time. Were an ideal intravenous anaesthetic agent to exist, it should have which of the following properties?

A. Produce recognizable symptoms on inadvertent arterial injection
B. Short shelf-life at room temperature
C. Not be an analgesic at subanaesthetic concentrations
D. Mainly ionized at physiological pH thus rapid onset
E. Have a water-soluble formulation

Question 19

Which of the following regarding temperature compensation of vaporizers is most accurate?

A. Vaporizers are insulated to maintain a constant temperature.
B. The Oxford miniature vaporizer incorporates a metal heat sink.
C. Temperature stabilization can be achieved with bimetallic strips.
D. Temperature compensation is not necessary for the TEC 6 vaporizer.
E. Most vaporizers incorporate a thermometer.

Question 20

A primiparous woman who is 30 weeks pregnant attends an anaesthetic antenatal clinic. Her foetus has intra-uterine growth restriction due to an abnormal placenta. Regarding the foetal and placental circulation, which of the following best describes the oxygen saturations in the ductus venosus, foetal ascending aorta and foetal descending aorta, respectively?

A. 80–90%, 60–65% and 55–60%
B. 50–55%, 40–45% and 30–35%
C. 60–65%, 50–55% and 55%
D. 100%, 85–90% and 70–75%
E. 80–85%, 75–80% and 70–75%

Question 21

Which is the most accurate statement about the intravenous anaesthetic agent thiopentone?

A. It acts by inhibiting gamma amino butyric acid (GABA).
B. It has analgesic activity.
C. It has a tocolytic effect on the uterus.
D. It has very low protein binding.
E. It is the sulphur analogue of the oxybarbiturate pentobarbitone.

Question 22

You are seconded to a hospital at 3000 m altitude. You intend to maintain anaesthesia with desflurane for an American Society of Anesthesiologists (ASA) physical status 2 patient undergoing an appendectomy using a circle system. Which of the following would you expect?

A. The dialled vapour concentration would need to be reduced.
B. TEC 5 vaporizers are most suitable.
C. Flow rates would need to be increased to compensate for lower ambient pressure.
D. A higher inspired concentration of oxygen would be required.
E. Low-flow anaesthesia is recommended.

Question 23

The ability of haemoglobin to carry more CO_2 in its deoxygenated state is referred to as

A. The chloride shift
B. The Bohr effect
C. The Haldane effect
D. Diffusion limitation
E. The second gas effect

Question 24

A group of anaesthetic trainees are discussing dose–response curves for routinely used anaesthetic drugs. They unanimously agree that agonists bind to a receptor with high affinity and a high intrinsic activity. However, they have a difference of opinion on the following statements. Which of the statements below is most correct?

A. A partial agonist has a high intrinsic activity but low affinity.
B. Competitive antagonists do not bind to receptors.
C. Phenoxybenzamine is a non-competitive antagonist.
D. Physiological antagonism of different receptors creates similar effects.
E. Allosteric modulators act on the agonist receptor.

Question 25

Spinal anaesthesia is the preferred method of anaesthesia for elective Caesarean section. When choosing a spinal needle type, which of the following statements is most relevant?

A. A 22-gauge needle is normally used.
B. The Whitacre needle has a 10% incidence of post-dural puncture headache.
C. The Sprotte needle has the side port closest to the needle tip.
D. The Quincke needle is short bevelled.
E. The Sprotte needle has a smaller side port than the Whitacre needle.

Question 26

A fit and well 28-year-old female ascends to an altitude of 2000 m above sea level. Which of the following would tend to oppose physiological adaptation to hypoxia at that altitude?

A. Hyperventilation-induced alkalaemia
B. Renal excretion of bicarbonate
C. Polycythaemia
D. Shift of the oxygen dissociation curve to the right
E. Increased plasma erythropoietin levels

Question 27

Second messengers like cyclic adenosine monophosphate (cAMP) link extracellular chemical signals (first messengers) to produce a physiological response intracellularly. Which of the following pairs is correctly matched?

A. Ion channel opening and closing: action of norepinephrine on K+ channels in the heart
B. mRNA transcription: insulin
C. Activation of phospholipase C: B1 receptor
D. Tyrosine kinase in cytoplasm: angiotensin II
E. Activation of adenylate cyclase: neuromuscular junction

Question 28

Which of the following statements regarding the desflurane vaporizer is true?

A. It is a plenum vaporizer.
B. It is heated to 42°C.
C. The vaporizer cannot be filled during use.
D. The saturated vapour pressure in the chamber is 100 kPa.
E. It is not temperature compensated.

Question 29

A 50-year-old patient with alcoholic liver disease undergoes a duplex ultrasound scan to estimate liver blood flow. Regarding liver blood supply in healthy individuals, which statement best describes the various contributions of the vessels involved?

A. 60% from hepatic artery and 40% from portal vein
B. 30% from hepatic artery and 70% from portal vein
C. 90% from hepatic artery and 10% from portal vein
D. Hepatic artery only
E. Portal vein only

Question 30

Which of the following statements best describes drug elimination?

A. Renal excretion is unaffected by glomerular filtration rate (GFR), water solubility and tubular secretion.
B. Most drugs follow zero-order kinetics during elimination.
C. A variable amount of drug elimination per unit time is called zero-order kinetics.
D. A constant amount of drug eliminated per unit time is caked first-order kinetics.
E. With saturation of elimination pathways, zero-order kinetics replaces first-order kinetics.

6 PAPER 3 ANSWERS

Answer 1: C

One volt (V) is defined as the potential difference across a segment of wire necessary to allow the flow of one ampere of current while there is dissipation of one watt of power.

The ampere (A) is a measure of current and is defined as the movement of one coulomb of charge (equivalent to 6.24×10^{18} electrons) past a point in one second.

The amount of current that can flow across a material at a given potential difference is determined by the resistance (R). Good conductors have low resistance, whereas insulators have high resistance. A thicker wire, having a higher cross-sectional area, has lower resistance.

Ohm's law links current, resistance and potential difference: $V = IR$.

The unit of power is the watt, or joules per second.

Further reading

Davies, P., and Kenny, G. *Basic Physics and Measurement in Anaesthesia*. 5th ed. London: Butterworth Heinemann, 2005.

Answer 2: C

Exercise induces many cardiac, respiratory, metabolic and physiological changes. These are partly mediated by the thought of exercise but also by physical activity via mechanoreceptors in muscle and joints, baroreceptors and local biochemical changes at the tissue level. Sympathetic tone increases, and parasympathetic tone decreases. Cardiac output increases (mediated by a tachycardia), and stroke volume (SV) changes little except in trained athletes. Both the systolic and diastolic blood pressures increase due to increased cardiac output. However, due to a decrease in systemic vascular resistance (SVR), the systolic rises more. Muscle activity acts as a mechanical pump and increases venous return, as does the effect of increased ventilation and the thoracic pump. There is increased blood flow to metabolizing muscle and to skin to maintain temperature. Blood flow is diverted from splanchnic and renal systems to meet the tissue demands of the heart and muscle. Coronary blood flow can increase up to five times compared to at rest. The oxygen dissociation curve moves to the right as a result of tissue acidosis and increased tissue $PaCO_2$. For detailed information, see the references given here.

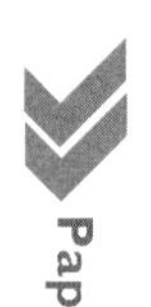
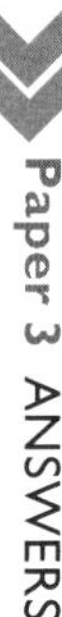

Further reading

Spoors, C., and Kiff, K. *Training in Anaesthesia: The Essential Curriculum*. Oxford: Oxford University Press, 2010, 226–7, 258.
Yentis, S., Hirsch, N., and Smith, G. *Anaesthesia and Intensive Care A–Z*. 4th ed. London: Churchill Livingstone, 2009.

Answer 3: C

Tautomerism is the ability of a molecule to undergo a change in molecular structure. Midazolam is a tautomer that can readily interconvert between a ring form and an open structure. At a pH below 4, it is ionized in solution and is found in an open structure, thus making it water soluble. At higher pH (e.g. in the plasma), it becomes unionized and a closed ring structure results. This makes the molecule lipid soluble and allows the drug to cross the blood–brain barrier.

Mivacurium contains geometric isomers (*trans-trans*, *cis-trans* and *cis-cis*), while S-ketamine is an enantiopure preparation.

Further reading

Peck, T.E., Williams, M., and Hill, S.A. *Pharmacology for Anaesthesia and Intensive Care*. Cambridge: Cambridge University Press, 2003.

Answer 4: C

Anemometry is the measurement of gas velocity. In hot-wire anemometry, a wire situated within a tube is heated to a fixed temperature. As gas flows over the hot wire, cooling occurs. The rate at which the wire cools is proportional to the square root of the gas velocity and as the wire cools, the resistance increases. The hot wire is incorporated into a Wheatstone bridge arrangement. In constant-temperature hot-wire anemometry, the output from the Wheatstone bridge is used as a feedback mechanism. The output is amplified and used to control the current passing through the wire to keep it at constant temperature. Hence, the output from the amplifier is a measure of gas velocity. Flow can be calculated as gas velocity × the cross-sectional area of the tube. The system requires calibration as heat transfer from the wire is dependent on the physical characteristics of gas. It is not suitable for use in gas containing flammable agents such as ethyl ether.

Further reading

Davey, A., and Diba, A. *Ward's Anaesthetic Equipment*. 5th ed. London: Elsevier Saunders, 2005.

Answer 5: C

The endothelial cell is a very underrated cell! It has many functions apart from proving a physical barrier between tissues and the vasculature. It governs tissue and blood exchange as it forms a selectively semipermeable membrane. It secretes vasoactive substances (nitric oxide [NO], prostacyclins and endothelins) in response to blood flow and can alter local blood flow. It plays an important role in haemostasis (or lack of) as the endothelium secretes prostacyclin which inhibits platelet aggregation and causes vasodilation. It plays an important role in the inflammatory process helping to guide and direct leukocytes to the affected area. Other roles include angiogenesis and an involvement in the pathogenesis of atheroma formation.

Further reading

Levick, J.R. *An Introduction to Cardiovascular Physiology*. 4th ed. London: Hodder Arnold, 2003, 131–48.

Answer 6: D

The mechanism of ion trapping can cause local anaesthetic toxicity in the foetus. Bupivacaine is most commonly used for epidural analgesia within the United Kingdom. In obstetrics, the foetus is relatively acidic compared to maternal pH, and if the foetal pH is reduced further in conditions like placental insufficiency (as in this case with foetal distress), then ion trapping can occur to cause foetal toxicity. As the pH falls more, bupivacaine will get ionized within the foetus and become trapped. Accumulation of this ionized fraction can result in toxicity. Inherited enzyme defect in the foetus can prevent breakdown of suxamethonium causing a prolonged depolarizing block at the foetal neuromuscular (NM) junction after a general anaesthetic.

Further reading

Peck, T.E., Williams, M., and Hill, S.A. *Pharmacology for Anaesthesia and Intensive Care*. Cambridge: Cambridge University Press, 2003.

Answer 7: C

Diffusion is the process by which a substance moves from an area of higher concentration to one of lower concentration. It is directly related to temperature, as more kinetic energy is present at higher temperatures. The rate of diffusion of a gas across a membrane is dependent on several other factors:

1. State of matter: liquid or gas.
2. Molecular size: Graham's Law states that the rate of diffusion is inversely proportional to the square root of the molecular weight.

3. Concentration gradient: Fick's Law states that the rate of diffusion is proportional to the concentration gradient across the membrane. The modified Fick's Law states that diffusion is proportional to the partial pressure.
4. Solubility coefficient: the solubility of a gas also affects the rate of diffusion. Carbon dioxide, being 20 times more soluble than oxygen, will diffuse faster than oxygen.
5. Membrane area and thickness: diffusion is directly proportional to the membrane area and inversely proportional to the membrane thickness.

Further reading

Yentis, S., Hirsch, N., and Smith, G. *Anaesthesia and Intensive Care A–Z.* 4th ed. London: Churchill Livingstone, 2009.

Answer 8: A

Pulmonary artery pressures are normally between 8 and 25 mmHg. Pulmonary vascular resistance (PVR) may be affected by many factors. PVR is typically increased by low PaO_2 (hypoxic pulmonary vasoconstriction), high $PaCO_2$, acidaemia, catecholamines, serotonin and histamine. PVR is decreased by low $PaCO_2$, high PaO_2, alkalaemia, acetylcholine, isoprenaline, volatile anaesthetics, prostacyclin and NO. PVR is also affected by intravascular pressures (cardiac output and venous pressures), lung volumes and the mechanical effect these have on the diameter of the pulmonary vasculature.

Further reading

Cross, M., and Plunkett, E. *Physics, Pharmacology and Physiology for Anaesthetists.* Cambridge: Cambridge University Press, 2008, 126.

Yentis, S., Hirsch, N., and Smith, G. *Anaesthesia and Intensive Care A–Z.* 4th ed. London: Churchill Livingstone, 2009.

Answer 9: B

Propofol is one of a number of drugs which may cause green urine. The propofol metabolite 4-glucoronide of 2,6 di-isopropylquinol produces the green colour. The renal function is not altered by this quinol. Other medications which may cause green urine include indomethacin and amitriptyline. Food dyes can also be excreted in the urine and change the colour of the urine. Furthermore, urinary tract infections, especially with *Pseudomonas* species, can give rise to green-tinged urine. Neither remifentanil esters nor catechol-O-methyltransferase (COMT) produces such effects.

Further reading

Shioya, N., Ishibe, Y., Shibata, S., Makabe, H., Kan, S., and Matsumoto, N. Green urine discoloration due to propofol infusion. *Case Rep Emerg Med* (2011): 242514.

Answer 10: D

The pertinent points in this scenario are that intubation is not possible and the patient requires urgent surgery. The Difficult Airway Society's 'can't incubate can't ventilate' algorithms should be followed. Help should be requested urgently. While help arrives, other airway devices can be used to oxygenate the patient. The best option in this situation would be to insert a laryngeal mask airway (LMA; e.g. a Proseal™ LMA, intubating LMA or the equivalent). If ventilation is possible, then it would be acceptable to proceed with surgery as this is a life-threatening situation. Attempts to secure the airway subsequently should be undertaken with expert assistance.

Further reading

Difficult Airway Society. Can't intubate, can't ventilate algorithm. http://www.das.uk.com/guidelines/downloads.html

Answer 11: D

Dead space is the volume of the lungs which does not take part in gaseous exchange either because it was not intended to (e.g. conducting airways) or because ventilated alveoli are not perfused. The former is called anatomical dead space, and the latter alveolar dead space. Physiological dead space = anatomical dead space + alveolar dead space.

In Fowler's method, an individual takes a single vital capacity breath of 100% O_2. Exhaled N_2 concentration is measured and plotted against time on the x-axis. Classically four phases of exhaled N_2 levels are seen: the first volumes of air exhaled are purely from the conducting airways, which will contain 100% O_2 and no N_2. The next phase will include a mixture of anatomical dead space volume and increasing component from alveolar gases, and thus the N_2 concentration will start to rise until it reaches a positively inclined plateau. This plateau corresponds to pure alveolar gas emptying. As the individual reaches closing capacity, there is a sudden upstroke in the N_2 concentration. For further detailed explanations, see the reference given here.

Further reading

Cross, M., and Plunkett, E. *Physics, Pharmacology and Physiology for Anaesthetists.* Cambridge: Cambridge University Press, 2008, 129.

Answer 12: C

Tachyphylaxis is defined as a rapid decrease in response to repeated doses of a drug over a short period of time. In this case, it occurs due to depletion of stores of transmitter. Ephedrine, an indirect sympathomimetic, relies on noradrenaline for its action. The synthesis of noradrenaline cannot meet the demands with its frequent ephedrine boluses, hence the refractory effect to ephedrine.

Desensitization is not an acute event, but instead it is a gradual loss of response to a drug used chronically. Desensitization is secondary to either a structural change in receptors or a reduced number of receptors.

Tolerance is the process whereby a larger dose is needed to produce a similar pharmacological effect (chronic opioid use).

Allosteric modulators alter the activity of a receptor without binding to the ligand-binding site. They act on sites distant to the ligand-binding site.

Antagonism alters the binding characteristics of the agonist.

Further reading

Peck, T.E., Williams, M., and Hill, S.A. *Pharmacology for Anaesthesia and Intensive Care*. Cambridge: Cambridge University Press, 2003.

Answer 13: A

Magnetic resonance imaging (MRI) scanners typically employ field strengths in the range of 0.5 to 3 Tesla. The Earth's magnetic field strength is typically 0.6 Gauss (I Tesla = 10 000 Gauss). The strong magnetic field is generated by a superconducting solenoid that is immersed in liquid helium maintained close to absolute zero. During an MRI, atoms with unpaired electrons (e.g. hydrogen and phosphorus) align with the magnetic field. Short bursts of radiofrequency energy are applied, which cause misalignment of atoms in relation to the magnetic field. When the radiofrequency pulse source is turned off, the atoms realign to the magnetic field. Realignment results in the release of low-frequency radiation which is detected and used to generate the image. The signal detected is very weak, and to prevent corruption by external radiofrequency sources, the MRI scanner is housed in a Faraday cage.

Further reading

Reddy, R., White, M.J., and Wilson, S.R. Anaesthesia for magnetic resonance imaging. *Contin Educ Anaesth Crit Care Pain* (2012) 12 (3): 140–144.

Stuart, G. Understanding magnetic resonance imaging. ATOTW 177. 2010. http://www.frca.co.uk/Documents/177%20Understanding%20Magnetic%20resonance%20imaging.pdf

Answer 14: A

Oxygen content of blood can be best estimated using the following equation:

Oxygen contained in blood in mL/L

= oxygen combined with Hb + oxygen dissolved in the plasma

= (Hb g/dL × 10 × saturations × 1.34 [Huffner constant]) + (PaO_2[kPa] × 10 × 0.0225mL O_2 dissolved per 100 mL plasma per kPa)

The principle behind this equation is that the greatest contribution to the arterial content of oxygen comes from the haemoglobin concentration and its saturations. PaO_2 makes little contribution.

Further reading

West, J.B. *Respiratory Physiology*. 7th ed. Philadelphia: Lippincott Williams and Wilkins, 2005, 75–80.

Yentis, S., Hirsch, N., and Smith, G. *Anaesthesia and Intensive Care A–Z*. 4th ed. London: Churchill Livingstone, 2009.

Answer 15: B

G proteins act as transducers creating a change within the cell from a stimulus outside the cell. In addition to conveying the stimulus, they also generate signal amplification across the cell membrane. G proteins can bind guanine diphosphate (GDP) and guanine triphosphate (GTP), hence the name 'G protein'. It has three subunits: α, β and γ. The inactive α GDP unit interacts with an active ligand receptor complex, and the GDP is replaced with a molecule of GTP to produce α GTPβγ unit. Subsequently, the α GTP dissociates from the complex and mediates an effect by activating or inhibiting effector proteins (adenyl cyclase or phospholipase C).

Further reading

Peck, T.E., Williams, M., and Hill, S.A. *Pharmacology for Anaesthesia and Intensive Care*. Cambridge: Cambridge University Press, 2003.

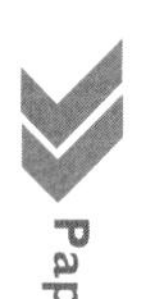

Answer 16: E

Careful assessment of the patient must be undertaken prior to MRI. Absolute contraindications to MRI include the presence of cochlear implants, intraocular metallic foreign bodies or shrapnel, or ferromagnetic clips, particularly in the neurovascular context. Patients with implanted pacemakers and defibrillators must be kept outside the 5 Gauss line, else these devices are likely to malfunction. In general, modern surgical prostheses are non-ferromagnetic and are safe in the scanner. Furthermore, sterna wires and general surgical clips and artificial valves are also deemed safe as they are fixed within fibrous tissue. The rapid switching of the gradient coils within the scanner produces high acoustic noise, often in excess of 85 decibels. Therefore, ear protection is mandatory for all patients. Protection may be delivered via ear plugs or via noise cancellation headsets. Oxygen sensors should be installed in the scanner as evaporation and leak of liquid helium, particularly during quenching, may produce a hypoxic environment if exhaust mechanisms are faulty. The safety of MRI during pregnancy remains a controversial subject. In general, it is best avoided in the first trimester of pregnancy.

Further reading

Stuart, G. Understanding magnetic resonance imaging. ATOTW 177. 2010. http://www.frca.co.uk/Documents/177%20Understanding%20Magnetic%20resonance%20imaging.pdf

Answer 17: D

A portal circulation is one which connects two capillary beds directly without going through the heart. Examples include the portal vein which links capillary beds in the gut and liver sinusoids, and the porto-hypophyseal circulation which connects the hypothalamic capillaries to the anterior pituitary capillaries.

Further reading

Ganong, W.F. *Review of Medical Physiology*. 22nd ed. New York: McGraw-Hill, 2005, 234, 624.

Answer 18: E

The ideal intravenous anaesthetic agent should act rapidly, be highly lipid soluble, have a rapid recovery profile, serve as an analgesic at subanaesthetic concentrations, cause no pain on injection and prove safe on accidental intra-arterial injection. It should also be water soluble and have a long shelf life at room temperature.

Further reading

Peck, T.E., Williams, M., and Hill, S.A. *Pharmacology for Anaesthesia and Intensive Care*. Cambridge: Cambridge University Press, 2003.

Answer 19: D

During anaesthesia, cooling of the vapour can occur for two reasons – first, the loss of the latent heat of vaporization; and, second, via changes in the ambient temperature. As the saturated vapour pressure is dependent on temperature, temperature regulation is crucial for accurate output. This can be achieved by two mechanisms. Vaporizers are constructed with built-in heat sinks with high heat capacities and thermal conductivity to equilibrate with the atmospheric temperature. This is known as temperature stabilization and is usually achieved with the incorporation of dense metals (plenum vaporizers). The Oxford miniature vaporizer utilizes glycol. Temperature compensation refers to the regulation of the fraction of gas flow through the vaporizer, so that the net output vapour concentration remains unchanged throughout anaesthesia. This is achieved by incorporating bimetallic strips or aneroid bellows (TEC series of vaporizers). The TEC 6 desflurane vaporizer is a measured flow vaporizer and does not require temperature compensatory mechanisms.

Further reading

Boumphrey, S., and Marshall, N. Understanding vaporisers. *Contin Educ Anaesth Crit Care Pain* (2012) 12 (6): 119–203.

Answer 20: A

The foetal and placental circulations are exam favourites, and you should know these in detail. Maternal blood reaching the placenta is 90–100% saturated. Some of this oxygen is used by the metabolic demands of the placenta. The foetal haemoglobin is left 80–90% saturated. This highly oxygenated blood passes through the ductus venosus and mixes with the venous return from the foetus (saturations of 25–40%) and travels into the right heart, where it is channelled by the christa terminalis and foramen ovale into the left heart and out of the ascending aorta at saturations of approximately 65%. This relatively highly oxygenated blood is sent preferentially, due to the nature of the foetal circulation, to the brain and upper part of the body. The descending aortal blood mixes with the blood returning from the superior vena cava via the ductus arteriosus to give saturations here of approximately 60% to the lower body. For a detailed explanation, please see the references given here.

Further reading

Spoors, C., and Kiff, K. *Training in Anaesthesia: The Essential Curriculum*. Oxford: Oxford University Press, 2010, 472–3.
Yentis, S., Hirsch, N., and Smith, G. *Anaesthesia and Intensive Care A–Z*. 4th ed. London: Churchill Livingstone, 2009.

Answer 21: E

Both benzodiazepines and barbiturates act by enhancing the inhibitory effects of the GABA (gamma amino butyric acid) receptor. However, unlike midazolam, barbiturates modulate the 'duration' of the GABA-dependent chloride channel opening and not the 'frequency'. The increased chloride transfer produces hyperpolarization and inhibits neurons. Thiopentone, unlike ketamine, has no analgesic activity. It has no effect on the uterus. It is 80% protein bound. It is the sulphur analogue of the oxybarbiturate pentobarbitone.

Further reading

Peck, T.E., Williams, M., and Hill, S.A. *Pharmacology for Anaesthesia and Intensive Care*. Cambridge: Cambridge University Press, 2003.

Answer 22: D

Desflurane has a boiling point close to room temperature and hence will require a metered dose vaporizer (TEC 6 vaporizer). This vaporizer chamber is at 2 atmospheres regardless of the ambient pressure, and when a percentage concentration is dialled, it delivers that concentration as a percentage of the ambient pressure. At an altitude of 3000 m, the ambient pressure is roughly 69 kPa. Hence, a lower partial pressure of desflurane would be present in the delivered output from the vaporizer. As the effect of a vapour is a function of its partial pressure, a higher dial setting should be dialled to maintain anaesthesia. Manufacturers provide tables of dialled concentration and output at different altitudes to correct for altitude use. To prevent hypoxia, a higher concentration of oxygen is often required at higher altitude (Dalton's Law of partial pressure). As at lower altitude, rotameters are not accurate unless calibrated, and low-flow anaesthesia is not recommended. Flow meters at higher altitude can under-read, and hence hypoxic mixtures can be delivered especially if nitrous oxide is concomitantly used.

Further reading

Davey, A., and Diba, A. *Ward's Anaesthetic Equipment*. 5th ed. London: Elsevier Saunders, 2005.

Davies, P., and Kenny, G. *Basic Physics and Measurement in Anaesthesia*. 5th ed. London: Butterworth Heinemann, 2005.

Answer 23: C

Diffusion limitation is a term applied to a gas whose uptake into the blood is dependent on factors affecting diffusion.

The second gas effect is a phenomenon seen when a volatile gas is administered with a high concentration of nitrous oxide.

The Haldane effect refers to the ability of haemoglobin to carry more CO_2 in its deoxygenated state.

The Bohr effect refers to the behaviour of the oxygen dissociation curve (right shift and increased O_2 off-loading) when exposed to conditions of a high $PaCO_2$, increased H+ and high temperatures.

CO_2 is carried in plasma and in red cells:

- In plasma, it is carried as a dissolved gas; $H_2O + CO_2 = H_2CO_3 = H+ + HCO_3-$, with the H+ being buffered in the plasma. This reaction is relatively slow due to the lack of carbonic anhydrase. CO_2 also forms carbamino compounds with plasma proteins.
- CO_2 is carried in the red cell combined with haemoglobin to form carbamino compounds, and as a dissolved gas as in the plasma, but here:
    1. The reaction is much quicker due to the presence of red cell carbonic anhydrase;
    2. The H+ produced is buffered by haemoglobin; and
    3. The HCO_3- produced moves out of the red cell (along its concentration gradient) into the plasma in exchange for Cl– to maintain electrical and chemical neutrality – this is the chloride shift.

Due to the Haldane effect, and the fact that haemoglobin is a better buffer of H+ in its deoxygenated state, the uptake of CO_2 in the red cell is promoted as red cells pass through capillaries, and thus the chloride shift is observed here. The chloride content of venous red blood cells is greater than in arterial red cells.

Further reading

Spoors, C., and Kiff, K. *Training in Anaesthesia: The Essential Curriculum*. Oxford: Oxford University Press, 2010, 357.

Ganong, W.F. *Review of Medical Physiology*. 22nd ed. New York: McGraw-Hill, 2005, 669–70.

Answer 24: C

A partial agonist has both high affinity and intrinsic activity. Competitive agonists have no direct effects. They do bind to agonist receptors reversibly. Opposing effects are produced by physiological antagonism of different receptors (e.g. histamine and adrenaline causing broncho-constriction and broncho-dilatation, respectively).

Phenoxybenzamine is a non-competitive antagonist.

Allosteric modulators alter the response of a receptor to a ligand without acting on the actual ligand site.

Further reading

Peck, T.E., Williams, M., and Hill, S.A. *Pharmacology for Anaesthesia and Intensive Care*. Cambridge: Cambridge University Press, 2003.

Answer 25: D

The shape of the needle tip and the gauge are important factors which affect the incidence of post-dural puncture headaches. The Quincke needle is a short-bevelled cutting needle and has the highest incidence of post-dural puncture headaches (PDPHs). Pencil-point needles were subsequently introduced to reduce this high incidence of PDPHs. The Sprotte needle has a tapered tip, with a proximal side port for injection of intra-thecal drugs. This design significantly reduced the incidence of PDPHs as the dural fibres were split apart rather than being cleaved, thus allowing for easier closure of the puncture site. Although the Sprotte needle reduced the incidence of PDPHs, it has a significant failure rate, which is related to the relatively large side port size placed fairly proximal to the tip. This resulted in accidental extra-thecal deposition of drugs. The Whitacre needle is also a pencil-point needle with the side port more distal and smaller. Such a design improved on the failure rates seen with the Sprotte. The size of the needle also plays an important point in PDPHs, and the larger the needle, the higher the incidence. Normally, a 26- or sometimes a 25-gauge needle is used for spinal anaesthesia. Modern 26-guage pencil-point needles have less than 1% incidence of PDPHs.

Further reading

Anaesthesia UK. Spinal anaesthesia: choice of needles. 2004. http://www.frca.co.uk/article.aspx?articleid=100127

Answer 26: A

Although FiO_2 remains unchanged, PaO_2 decreases with altitude as atmospheric pressure decreases. This hypoxic stimulation causes short-term and long-term physiological changes enabling the individual to adapt. Peripheral chemoreceptor stimulation causes an increase in minute volume and alveolar ventilation – this also results in a hypocapnia which, according to the alveolar gas equation, will increase the PaO_2. The hyperventilation also causes a respiratory alkalosis and an alkalaemia. The reduced $PaCO_2$ also acts to reduce the amount of dissolved H+ in cerebrospinal fluid (CSF) and blood which would tend to oppose any further increases in minute volume. However, this itself is prevented from happening due to three mechanisms:

1. Active transport of bicarbonate out of the CSF by the choroid plexus;
2. Renal excretion of the additional bicarbonate; and
3. Re-setting of the respiratory centre sensitivities.

Renal erythropoietin secretion is stimulated within 2 hours of hypoxia at altitude and serves to stimulate the production of red cells, but the increase in haemoglobin is seen 3–5 days later. This adaptation allows the blood to increase its oxygen content and hence oxygen delivery.

Further reading

Power, I., and Kam, P. *Principles of Physiology for the Anaesthetist*. 2nd ed. London: Hodder Arnold, 2008, 432–4.
Spoors, C., and Kiff, K. *Training in Anaesthesia: The Essential Curriculum*. Oxford: Oxford University Press, 2010, 366–7.

Answer 27: A

- Ion channel opening and closing: action of norepinephrine on K+ channels in the heart and NM junction
- mRNA transcription: thyroid hormones and steroid hormones
- Activation of phospholipase C: angiotensin II and alpha 2 receptor
- Tyrosine kinase in cytoplasm: insulin
- Activation of adenylate cyclase: B_1 receptor

Further reading

Peck, T.E., Williams, M., and Hill, S.A. *Pharmacology for Anaesthesia and Intensive Care*. Cambridge: Cambridge University Press, 2003.

Answer 28: E

As desflurane has a boiling point close to room temperature (22.6°C), its saturated vapour pressure varies unpredictably, thus making plenum vaporizers unsuitable for delivery. Desflurane requires a specially designed measured-flow vaporizer. The chamber of the vaporizer is heated to a temperature of 39°C, which results in a desflurane vapour pressure of 200 kPa. The vapour is injected into the fresh gas flow, and a differential pressure transducer is incorporated into the system to allow the electronic control of the amount of agent injected. It is very accurate at low flow rates. The vaporizer requires an electrical source (mains or battery) and a warm-up time (5–10 minutes), and can be filled while in use.

Further reading

Davies, P., and Kenny, G. *Basic Physics and Measurement in Anaesthesia*. 5th ed. London: Butterworth Heinemann, 2005.
Davey, A., and Diba, A. *Ward's Anaesthetic Equipment*. 5th ed. London: Elsevier Saunders, 2005.

Answer 29: B

The blood supply of the liver arises from two sources:

1. The hepatic artery, which contributes 30%; and
2. The portal venous, which contributes 70%.

Both the arterial and venous blood contributes to the oxygen demands of the liver. The arterial blood, being 98% saturated, contributes around 30–40% of the oxygen requirements of the liver, with the portal vein (having drained the stomach, gallbladder, intestines, spleen and pancreas) having saturations around 85% and contributing the rest.

Further reading

Power, I., and Kam, P. *Principles of Physiology for the Anaesthetist.* 2nd ed. London: Hodder Arnold, 2008, 214–15.

Spoors, C., and Kiff, K. *Training in Anaesthesia: The Essential Curriculum.* Oxford: Oxford University Press, 2010, 434–5.

Answer 30: E

The glomerular filtration rate (GFR), water solubility and amount of secreted and absorbed drug affect the renal excretion of substances. Most drugs are eliminated by first-order kinetics whereby rate of elimination is proportional to the amount of drug remaining in the body. In zero-order kinetics, a constant amount of drug is eliminated per unit time (e.g. alcohol). At higher drug concentrations when elimination pathways are saturated, zero-order kinetics may replace first-order kinetics.

Further reading

Peck, T.E., Williams, M., and Hill, S.A. *Pharmacology for Anaesthesia and Intensive Care.* Cambridge: Cambridge University Press, 2003.

PAPER 4 QUESTIONS

Question 1

A marathon runner completes a 26-mile race and is estimated to finish the race in 3 hours. During the last few miles, which of the following muscle types is least likely to show signs of fatigue?

A. Smooth muscle of gut
B. Smooth muscle of the bladder
C. Myocardiocytes
D. Skeletal slow-type fibres
E. Skeletal fast-type fibres

Question 2

A 30-year-old female has had a laparoscopic cholecystectomy under general anaesthesia. Intraoperative analgesia was provided with fentanyl, morphine and local anaesthetic infiltration. In the recovery area, the patient complained of isolated right shoulder tip pain. There were no abdominal symptoms. The Senior House Officer (SHO) was asked by the registrar to prescribe a non-steroidal anti-inflammatory drug (NSAID) from the pyrrole group. Which of the following drug is an appropriate choice?

A. Aspirin
B. Diclofenac
C. Ibuprofen
D. Piroxicam
E. Ketorolac

Question 3

Which of the following statements regarding capacitors is true?

A. They consist of a metal plate inserted between two dielectrics.
B. The amount of charge stored is inversely proportional to the voltage.
C. Capacitors are not required in modern defibrillators.
D. Capacitance is the ability of an object to hold current.
E. Capacitance can be expressed as coulomb per volt.

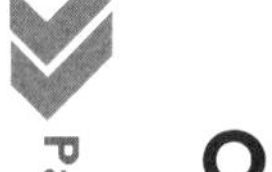

Question 4

A medical student is shown the histological cross-sections of human capillaries. A fenestrated capillary endothelium is most likely to be seen in which of the following organs?

A. Myocardium
B. Kidney
C. Lungs
D. Brain
E. Liver

Question 5

A 20-year-old man has presented for emergency repair of torsion of the testis. He is fit and well but is allergic to suxamethonium. He had lunch 4 hours ago. A modified rapid sequence induction with rocuronium is planned. Which of the following best describes rocuronium?

A. Chemically related to vecuronium.
B. Does not exhibit fade and post-tetanic potentiation.
C. Duration of action shortened by hypokalaemia.
D. Muscle relaxation produced by allosteric inhibition and not antagonism.
E. Neostigmine is its only reversal agent.

Question 6

Which of the following statements regarding a defibrillator is incorrect?

A. A step-down transformer is located in the charging circuit.
B. The rectifier is located in the charging circuit.
C. The inductor is located in the discharging circuit.
D. The rectifier converts alternating current to direct current.
E. During charging, the potential difference across the capacitor exceeds 5000 volts.

Question 7

Following glomerular filtration in a dehydrated patient, water and salts are re-absorbed into the renal parenchyma from the loop of Henle via which of the following means?

A. Afferent arteriole
B. Efferent arteriole
C. Vasa recta
D. Peritubular capillaries
E. Renal vein

Question 8

A 55-year-old man is admitted on the intensive therapy unit (ITU) with community-acquired pneumonia. Over the next 24 hours he becomes septic, needing haemodynamic support. His past medical history includes non-insulin-dependent diabetes mellitus (NIDDM) and ischaemic heart disease. Inotropes that target adrenergic receptors were chosen to provide haemodynamic support. Adrenergic receptors are also found in non-vascular tissue. Which of the following would be an appropriate response of stimulating the stated adrenergic receptor?

A. Intestinal α-1 receptors: smooth muscle contraction with relaxation of sphincters
B. Pancreatic α-1 receptors: secretion of insulin, glucagon and pancreatic enzymes
C. α-2 receptors on platelets: inhibits aggregation of platelets
D. β-1 receptors in kidney: inhibits renin formation
E. β-2 receptors in liver: breakdown of glycogen

Question 9

Which of the following statements regarding the generation and supply of electricity is incorrect?

A. The generator incorporates magnets.
B. In the United Kingdom, the peak mains voltage is 240 V.
C. Substations incorporate step-down transformers.
D. The neutral wire is earthed at the substation.
E. Current flows back to the substation via the neutral wire.

Question 10

An intravenously (IV) administered marker of plasma clearance is given to a patient. Its plasma concentration is found to be 0.5 mg/mL. Its urine concentration is found to be 5 mg/mL. Which other variable would you find most useful when calculating the clearance of this marker?

A. Urine volume in mL
B. Urine flow in mL/min
C. Water content of the blood
D. Glomerular filteration rate (GFR)
E. Dose of marker administered in mg

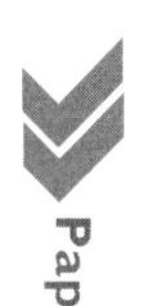

Question 11

Drugs which produce the effects of stimulation of the parasympathetic nervous system are called *parasympathomimetic drugs*. Which of the following is a parasympathomimetic drug?

A. Drugs which inhibit acetylcholine receptors like acetylcholine
B. Synthetic choline esters like pilocarpine
C. Acetyl cholinesterase inhibitors
D. Cholimimetic alkaloids like carbachol
E. Dopamine

Question 12

Which of the following statements regarding saturated vapour pressure is true?

A. It is the pressure exerted when a liquid boils.
B. It increases with increasing surface area.
C. It is related to temperature.
D. It cannot equal ambient pressure.
E. It increases at higher altitude.

Question 13

Which of the following mechanisms would be least useful to increase the GFR of a normal kidney?

A. Constriction of the afferent arteriole
B. Vasodilation of the afferent arteriole
C. Vasoconstriction of the efferent arteriole
D. Increasing plasma oncotic pressure
E. Increasing renal blood flow

Question 14

The volume of distribution (Vd) is the volume of water that an injected dose will have to dilute to, in order to equate the measured plasma concentration. Which other statement of the Vd given here is most accurate?

A. If the Vd equals total body water volume, then the drug is confined to plasma.
B. If the Vd equals blood volume, then the drug is distributed equally throughout the body.
C. If the Vd is less than total body water volume, then the drug is concentrated in the tissues.
D. Drugs with a small Vd are more easily cleared from the plasma by haemodialysis.
E. Drugs with a large Vd, once cleared from the plasma, have no recurrent toxicity.

Question 15

Choose the correct statement regarding the physical properties of inhalational vapour used in anaesthesia.

A. A high boiling point is desirable for an ideal agent.
B. The minimum alveolar concentration value is proportional to the oil–gas partition coefficient.
C. Potency is a function of lipid solubility.
D. Quick emergence occurs when the blood–gas solubility is relatively high.
E. Onset of effect is slow when blood–gas solubility is low.

Question 16

A 26-year-old cyclist is brought into the accident and emergency (A&E) resuscitation department following a collision with a lorry. He has a heart rate of 160 and blood pressure of 69/38 mmHg and is bleeding from a wound to the right flank. In haemorrhage, which of the following mechanisms is unlikely to be responsible for the release of aldosterone?

A. Plasma potassium concentration
B. Sympathetic stimulation
C. Anxiety
D. Hyponatraemia
E. Anti-diuretic hormone

Question 17

The Vd has been measured for several drugs that have been administered to a patient on the intensive care unit. Which value for Vd is most precisely paired with the respective drug?

A. Digoxin: 9 L
B. Insulin: 50 L
C. Lignocaine: 500 L
D. Propranolol: 12 L
E. Aspirin: 250 L

Question 18

Which of the following regarding the colligative properties of solutions is true?

A. The freezing point of a solvent is increased by the presence of solute.
B. Osmolality is defined as the number of osmotically active particles per kilogram of solvent.
C. Decreasing osmolality increases the boiling point.
D. Raoult's Law states that increasing osmolality increases the vapour pressure of the solvent.
E. Tonicity is the oncotic pressure of a colloid.

Question 19

A 28-year-old trauma patient sustained a fracture and spinal cord transection at the T9 level. Having spent a long time on the ITU, he is currently in community rehabilitation. He is unable to walk and mobilizes in a wheelchair. He has developed sepsis from an infected pressure sore on his coccygeal area and needs urgent debridement. An exaggerated response to depolarizing muscle relaxants in this patient would be due to which one of the following?

A. Pre-junctional acetylcholine receptors
B. Extra-junctional acetylcholine receptors
C. Post-junctional acetylcholine receptors
D. Decreased levels of acetylcholine-esterase
E. Antibodies to acetylcholine receptors

Question 20

A medical representative from a colloid-producing company is delivering a luncheon. She mentions that their company manufactures albumin, hetastarch, pentastarch, gelatine derivatives and dextrans. While presenting a pro–con debate in favour of her products over crystalloids, she states the following. Which of the statements presented is untrue?

A. Colloids do not traverse a semipermeable membrane.
B. Colloids are initially confined to the intravascular compartment.
C. Colloids are useful in temporarily replacing vascular volumes (e.g. haemorrhage).
D. Colloids are more useful in correcting specific water and electrolyte deficiencies.
E. Colloids expand plasma volume due to their high osmolality.

Question 21

Which of the following statements regarding diathermy is correct?

A. Current flows from the active plate to the neutral plate.
B. Typically a current with high frequency (e.g. 1000 MHz) is used.
C. The neutral pad should be of large area and placed away from the chest when using bipolar diathermy.
D. Coagulation is optimal when a pulsed sine wave pattern-alternating current is used.
E. Monopolar diathermy is contraindicated when a pacemaker is *in situ*.

Question 22

50 mL of a strongly acidic solution is accidently given via IV to a patient. Which of the body's mechanisms is first to react to deal with this insult?

A. An increase in the respiratory rate
B. Increased renal excretion of hydrogen
C. Decreased renal excretion and increased reabsorption of bicarbonate
D. Extracellular buffer systems
E. Extracellular and intracellular buffer systems

Question 23

Which of the following statements regarding carbon dioxide absorbers is most accurate?

A. Baralyme is superior to soda lime in its ability to absorb CO_2.
B. Reaction of soda lime with CO_2 is endothermic.
C. Barium hydroxide is the main constituent in baralyme.
D. Constituents are packed with silica to form a 4–8 mesh size.
E. Absorbers also scavenge nitrous oxide.

Question 24

A supine anaesthetized patient has been breathing 100% oxygen at tidal volume through a closed circuit for 60 minutes. FiO_2 is 99% and FeO_2 is 94%. Which of the following methods can be used to best increase the oxygen reserve of this patient?

A. Increasing the respiratory rate
B. Increasing tidal volume
C. Increasing the O_2 flow rate from 10 to 12 L/min
D. Increasing the functional respiratory capacity
E. Paralyzing the patient

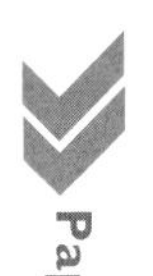

Question 25

A 5-month-old infant has been brought to the A&E department with a history of fever, decreased oral intake and irritability. His baseline investigations showed a remarkable electrocardiogram (ECG) with a rate of 220 per min, narrow QRS complexes and no P-waves. His femoral pulses are palpable, and he has a respiratory rate of 50 per min. Which of the following is the most appropriate initial step in management?

A. IV verapamil slow bolus.
B. IV adenosine fast bolus.
C. Apply an ice-filled plastic bag to the forehead for 5 seconds.
D. Transcutaneous cardiac pacing.
E. 2 J/Kg of synchronized direct current (DC) shock.

Question 26

With regards to medical gas cylinders, which of the statements below is most true?

A. Molybdenum steel cylinders should not be filled in excess of 150 bar pressure.
B. Composite cylinders are frequently found in the hospital setting.
C. Cylinders composed of aluminium are not strong enough for medical gases.
D. A size D cylinder holds 340 L of oxygen at 68.5 bar pressure.
E. The filling ratio of nitrous oxide in the United Kingdom is 0.67.

Question 27

A 50-year-old patient is admitted with a severe pulmonary oedema secondary to mitral valve disease. He is breathing 35% oxygen via a venturi mask, and his PaO_2 is 7.5 kPa with saturations of 89%. A chest radiograph shows significant basal collapse. How can his shunt fraction be improved best?

A. Increase FiO_2 to 55%.
B. Increase his cardiac output.
C. Apply CPAP.
D. Lie him in the supine position.
E. Give two units of blood to increase his haemoglobin.

Question 28

During pre-assessment of a pregnant woman in the antenatal clinic, the woman wants to know the toxicity and teratogenicity of drugs. Which of the following is correctly paired?

A. Sulphonamides: grey baby syndrome
B. Tetracycline: tooth enamel dysplasia and bone growth inhibition
C. Chloramphenicol: kernicterus

D. Valproic acid: ototoxicity
E. Streptomycin: neural tube defects

Question 29

Regarding rotameters, which of the following is most true?

A. Pressure changes proportionally with increasing flow rates.
B. It is calibrated to be read from the middle of the bobbin.
C. Needle valves will give rise to inaccuracies if placed proximally.
D. They are accurate to 2% of the true flow.
E. At low flow rates, gas flow is turbulent.

Question 30

A 10-year-old girl visits the emergency department with her mum. She is known to have mild asthma for which she uses her salbutamol inhaler three times a week. Her current symptoms are occasional nocturnal cough that wakes her up, and on auscultation there are signs of diffuse wheeze on expiration. She has no accessory muscle use, and her SpO_2 on room air is 95%. Which of the following is the best treatment for her now?

A. Nebulized salbutamol
B. Subcutaneous epinephrine
C. IV steroids
D. Nebulized cromolyn sodium
E. Oxygen via nasal cannula

PAPER 4 ANSWERS

Answer 1: C

Of the three types of muscle in the body, cardiac muscle is the most physiologically adapted to resist fatigue. Cardiac muscle contains relatively more mitochondria than smooth and skeletal muscle types and, unlike the other two types, it does not exhibit tetany.

Skeletal slow fibres are involved in prolonged contractions such as those needed to maintain posture and utilize aerobic metabolism.
Skeletal fast fibres are known as twitch fibres and are designed for infrequently required but intense action; they utilize anaerobic metabolism.

Further reading

Clifton, B., Armstrong S., et al. *Primary FRCA in a Box*. London: The Royal Society of Medicine Press Ltd, 2007, card 70.
Spoors, C., and Kiff, K. *Training in Anaesthesia: The Essential Curriculum*. Oxford: Oxford University Press, 2010, 213.

Answer 2: E

Non-steroidal anti-inflammatory drugs (NSAIDs) are classified into:

1. Salicylic acids: aspirin;
2. Propionic acids: ibuprofen, naproxen;
3. Acetic acids: diclofenac, indomethacin;
4. Fenamates: mefanamic acid, flufenamic acid;
5. Pyrazolones: phenylbutazone, azapropazone;
6. Oxicams: piroxicam, tenoxicam;
7. Pyrroles: ketorolac; and
8. COX-2 inhibitors: rofecoxib.

Further reading

Peck, T.E., Williams, M., and Hill, S.A. *Pharmacology for Anaesthesia and Intensive Care*. Cambridge: Cambridge University Press, 2003.

Answer 3: E

Capacitance is the ability of an object to hold a charge (current is movement of a charge past a point). The unit of capacitance is the Farad, which can be expressed as one coulomb per volt. A capacitor is an essential component of a defibrillator and is made of two conducting metal plates separated by a material (dielectric) that prevents current flow through the capacitor. The amount of charge that a capacitor is able to hold is directly proportional to the battery voltage, and furthermore when the capacitor is fully charged, the potential difference across it is the same as in the source battery. The amount of energy (E) a capacitor is able to store is related to the amount of stored charge, the capacitance and the potential difference across it, and is given by this formula:

$$E = 1/2\ CV^2$$

Further reading

Davies, P., and Kenny, G. *Basic Physics and Measurement in Anaesthesia*. 5th ed. London: Butterworth Heinemann, 2005.

Answer 4: B

The structure of endothelium varies according to the organ it is within and the functions required of it. Junctions between endothelial cells provide one mechanism of transport across an endothelial barrier, as do endocytosis and exocytosis. Alternatively, some capillaries are fenestrated. This means there are points in the endothelial cell where the cytoplasm is deficient and gaps in the endothelial cell are formed. Such fenestrated endothelium exists in the kidney, intestinal villi and some endocrine glands. Gaps can also be seen between endothelial cells as in the liver sinusoids. These gaps and fenestrations in turn may be spanned by membranes which serve to selectively allow the passage of particular substances.

Further reading

Ganong, W.F. *Review of Medical Physiology*. 22nd ed. New York: McGraw-Hill, 2005, 577–80.

Answer 5: A

Both rocuronium and vecuronium, being non-depolarizing neuromuscular blockers, exhibit fade and post-tetanic potentiation. They are chemically related and they work by competitively antagonizing acetylcholine at the neuromuscular junction. This non-depolarizing block can be enhanced by hypermagnesaemia, hypocalcaemia, myasthenia gravis and myasthenic syndrome and aminoglycoside antibiotics. Neostigmine displaces the muscle relaxant from the receptor, thus facilitating muscle contraction, whereas the newer reversal 'sugammadex' binds to neuromuscular blocking agents like rocuronium and vecuronium to form

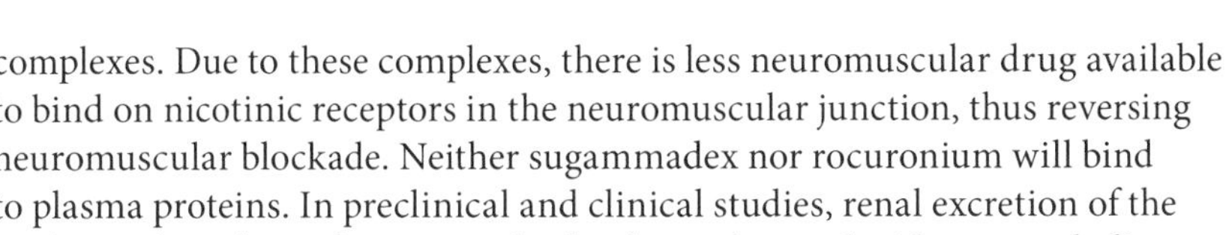

complexes. Due to these complexes, there is less neuromuscular drug available to bind on nicotinic receptors in the neuromuscular junction, thus reversing neuromuscular blockade. Neither sugammadex nor rocuronium will bind to plasma proteins. In preclinical and clinical studies, renal excretion of the unchanged product of sugammadex has been observed with no metabolites.

Further reading

Peck, T.E., Williams, M., and Hill, S.A. *Pharmacology for Anaesthesia and Intensive Care*. Cambridge: Cambridge University Press, 2003.

Answer 6: A

The defibrillator can be divided into two circuits. A step-up transformer is located in the charging circuit and generates potentials in excess of 5000 V from a mains voltage of 240 V to charge the capacitor. A rectifier incorporated into this circuit allows for an alternating current (AC) to be converted to direct current (DC). An AC is unable to charge the capacitor as the alternating nature results in charging and discharging at the plates. The capacitor is a key constituent and stores energy which is to be discharged to the patient. During discharge, a switch creates a discharging circuit, which connects the capacitor to the patient. It is at this time that energy is transferred from the capacitor to the myocardium. In order to limit the amount of energy delivered (for protection of the myocardium) and to prolong the time of current flow (increased success of cardioverting), an inductor is incorporated into the discharging circuit.

Further reading

Singh, S.K., Ingham, R., and Golding, J.P. Basics of electricity for anaesthetists. *Cont Educ Anaesth Crit Care Pain* (2012) 11 (6): 224–8.

Answer 7: C

The renal circulation is best understood by starting with the renal artery. This branches into interlobar arteries, and then into arcuate arteries passing along the boundary between the cortex and medulla. Interlobular arteries branch at 90° angles from the arcuate arteries, and afferent arterioles (which go on to form glomerular capillaries) are branches of these. The glomerular capillaries drain into the efferent arteriole. These in turn give rise to peritubular capillaries which surround the renal tubular apparatus. The efferent arteries of the inner one-third of the cortex additionally provide capillaries which loop in and out of the medulla alongside the loop of Henle and collecting tubules – these are the vasa recta. Both the vasa recta and the renal peritubular capillaries drain to the renal vein.

Further reading

Lote, C.J. *Principles of Renal Physiology*. 4th ed. Dordrecht, the Netherlands: Kluwer Academic, 2000, 27–8.

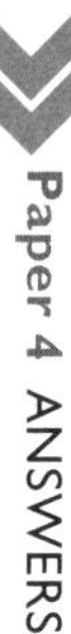

Answer 8: E

β-2 receptors in the liver, when stimulated, aid in glycogenolysis. The β-1 receptors in the renal juxtaglomerular apparatus promote renin secretion. α-1 receptors in the gut relax the intestinal smooth muscle and contract the sphincters, while the pancreatic α-1 receptors inhibit pancreatic hormones (insulin and glucagon) and enzymes production. Stimulating the α-2 receptors aggregates platelets.

Further reading

Peck, T.E., Williams, M., and Hill, S.A. *Pharmacology for Anaesthesia and Intensive Care*. Cambridge: Cambridge University Press, 2003.

Answer 9: B

Electricity is produced when turbines, powered by water or steam, cause a magnet housed in the generator to spin within coils of wire. This motion of the magnet causes movement of electrons with the wire, thereby producing electricity. The very high voltages (16 kV) produced in the power station are reduced to mains voltages by step-down transformers housed at substations. In the United Kingdom, the peak voltage is 340 V. However, this voltage varies in a sine wave fashion because of the alternating nature of the current. To relate this to DC, the root mean square (RMS) of AC is used and in the United Kingdom this is 240 V; a 240 RMS voltage of AC has the same heating effect and energy production as a 240 V DC.

Electricity flows from the substation to the equipment via the live wire and returns via the neutral wire. The neutral wire is also connected to earth at the substation.

Further reading

Singh, S.K., Ingham, R., and Golding, J.P. Basics of electricity for anaesthetists. *Cont Educ Anaesth Crit Care Pain* (2012) 11 (6): 224–8.

Answer 10: B

Renal clearance of a substance is defined as the volume of plasma from which the substance is completely removed in mL/min. The equation to calculate this is as follows:

Clearance (mL/min) = urine concentration of substance urine (mg/mL) × urine flow (mL/min) / concentration of substance in the plasma (mg/mL)

Inulin is a substance which is neither secreted nor reabsorbed once filtered by the kidney. Thus, its clearance can be used to measure the glomerular filtration rate (GFR).

Para-aminohippuric acid is a substance which is filtered and secreted by the kidney, and thus the clearance of this can be used to measure renal blood flow (Fick's Law).

Further reading

Lote, C.J. *Principles of Renal Physiology*. 4th ed. Dordrecht, the Netherlands: Kluwer Academic, 2000, 86–8.

Answer 11: C

Parasympathomimetic drugs mimic acetylcholine and produce a cholinergic response. Acetylcholine has diffuse actions and therefore is not used therapeutically. Pilocarpaine is a cholinergic alkaloid used in ophthalmology to treat glaucoma. Carbachol is a synthetic choline ester and acts on both nicotinic and muscarinic receptors. It is commonly used to treat glaucoma and urinary retention. Acetyl cholinesterase inhibitors like neostigmine produce parasympathetic effects. Dopamine is a sympathomimetic.

Further reading

Peck, T.E., Williams, M., and Hill, S.A. *Pharmacology for Anaesthesia and Intensive Care*. Cambridge: Cambridge University Press, 2003.

Answer 12: C

Within a closed system containing a liquid, thermodynamic equilibrium between the liquid and vapour phase occurs. The pressure exerted by the vapour phase at equilibrium is referred to as the *saturated vapour pressure* (SVP). This pressure is dependent exclusively on temperature; SVP increases and decreases with temperature. Therefore, SVP for a substance is stated at a particular temperature. The temperature at which the SVP of a liquid equals the ambient temperature is known as the *boiling point*. For a given temperature, SVP remains the same despite changes in ambient pressure, for example as a result of high altitude. However, the liquid will boil at lower temperatures as ambient pressure is reduced.

Further reading

Simpson, S. Vaporisers. *Update Anaesthes* (2002) (14): Article 16. http://www.nda.ox.ac.uk/wfsa/html/u14/u1416_01.htm

Answer 13: A

GFR is defined as the rate of fluid and solute filtration across the glomerular membrane and occurs across the fenestrated renal capillaries. The rate at which filtration occurs depends on the pressure gradient across the glomerulus and renal blood flow.

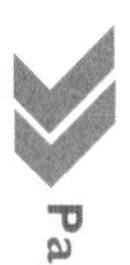

Filtration dynamics depend on a similar principle to Starling's forces which govern flow across a capillary. Changes in the hydrostatic pressure gradient across the glomerulus will affect the GFR such that, if it is increased by virtue of vasodilation of the afferent arteriole, GFR will increase. Vasoconstriction of the efferent arteriole is most likely to have the same effect. Vasoconstriction of the afferent arteriole will decrease renal blood flow. Increased hydrostatic pressure in the renal tubules (from severe obstructive uropathy) will tend to oppose the flow of fluid and substances out of the glomerular capillaries and reduce GFR.

Further reading

Lote, C.J. *Principles of Renal Physiology*. 4th ed. Dordrecht, the Netherlands: Kluwer Academic, 2000, 37–44, 92–5.

Answer 14: D

If Vd = blood volume, then the drug is restricted to the plasma.
If Vd = total body water volume, then the drug is equally distributed throughout the body.
If Vd > total body water, then the drug is concentrated in the tissues.
Drugs with a small Vd are easily cleared from the plasma by haemodialysis or haemofiltration. Those with a large Vd may be cleared from the plasma, but levels can rise again once the patient is off renal replacement therapy.

Further reading

Peck, T.E., Williams, M., and Hill, S.A. *Pharmacology for Anaesthesia and Intensive Care*. Cambridge: Cambridge University Press, 2003.

Answer 15: C

Potency is the measure of the ability of a drug to generate an action. It is usually expressed as the amount of drug needed to produce a predetermined effect. The minimum alveolar concentration (MAC) is a measure of potency and correlates with the oil–gas partition (i.e. volatile agents that have reduced lipid solubility are less potent) (the Meyer–Overton hypothesis). The speed of onset is determined by the solubility of the vapour in the blood. A vapour with a high blood–gas partition coefficient has a slower onset of action. This is because the blood and tissues act as a sink for vapour. Furthermore, large amounts of vapour will accumulate in the blood and tissues over time, and delay emergence. A high boiling point for a vapour would indicate difficulties in vapourization and would not be advantageous.

Further reading

Fenton, P. Volatile anaesthetic agents. *Update Anaesthes* (2000) (11): Article 15. http://www.nda.ox.ac.uk/wfsa/html/u11/u1115_01.htm

Answer 16: E

Aldosterone is a steroid hormone produced by the zona glomerulosa of the adrenal glands. Its release is triggered by four main routes:

1. Adrenocorticotrophic hormone (ACTH);
2. Plasma K concentration (hyperkalaemia);
3. The renin–angiotensin system (also activated by sympathetic stimulation); and
4. Hyponatraemia (which has a direct effect on the adrenal gland).

Aldosterone serves to promote sodium reabsorption from urine, from salivary secretions and in sweat glands. In the distal convoluted tubule and the collecting ducts, it serves to increase the absorption of sodium and water at the expense of potassium and hydrogen ions. Antidiuretic hormone, although likely to be present in high concentrations during the physiological response to haemorrhage, is not known to stimulate the secretion of aldosterone. Body fluid and electrolyte regulation are closely tied together, and changes in one affect the other.

Further reading

Power, I., and Kam, P. *Principles of Physiology for the Anaesthetist*. 2nd ed. London: Hodder Arnold, 2008, 238–44, 345–6.

Yentis, S., Hirsch, N., and Smith, G. *Anaesthesia and Intensive Care A–Z*. 4th ed. London: Churchill Livingstone, 2009.

Answer 17: B

Examples of a Vd are as follows: digoxin: 500 L; insulin: 50 L; lignocaine: 120 L; propranolol: 250 L; aspirin: 12 L; and warfarin: 9 L.

Further reading

Peck, T.E., Williams, M., and Hill, S.A. *Pharmacology for Anaesthesia and Intensive Care*. Cambridge: Cambridge University Press, 2003.

Answer 18: B

Osmolality is defined as the number of osmotically active particles in a kilogram of solvent. Osmolarity, on the other hand, is the number of osmotically active particles in 1 L of solvent. The addition of solutes to a solvent affects both the freezing and boiling points of the solvent. The higher the concentration of solutes, the higher the boiling point and the lower the freezing point. The depression of the freezing point is exploited by the osmometer which is used to measure osmolarity. The vapour pressure exerted by the solvent is depressed with increasing solute (Raoult's Law). The tonicity of a solution compares the effective osmotic pressure of the fluid with plasma when the solution is given intravenously. For example, 5% glucose is isosmotic to plasma. Once infused, however, the glucose is removed to liberate free water. Hence, 5% dextrose is hypotonic as free water has no osmotic pressure.

Further reading

Yentis, S., Hirsch, N., and Smith, G. *Anaesthesia and Intensive Care A–Z*. 4th ed. London: Churchill Livingstone, 2009.

Answer 19: B

Nicotinic post-junctional receptors are present at the post-junctional membrane of the neuromuscular junction and are necessary for normal neuromuscular transmission to occur. Pre-junctional receptors are present on the pre-junctional neuromuscular membrane and have a role in 'fade' phenomena seen with nondepolarizing neuromuscular blockade. Extra-junctional nicotinic receptors proliferate in denervation injuries and in burns patients and are located along the muscle membrane. The worry in these circumstances is that when these extra-junctional acetylcholine receptors are stimulated by depolarizing muscle relaxants, a massive efflux of potassium will ensue from the muscle cell - enough to precipitate a cardiac arrest. Decreased levels of acetylcholine-esterase are not typically seen in such injuries. Antibodies to acetylcholine receptors are seen in myasthenia gravis.

Further reading

Anaesthesia UK. The neuromuscular junction. http://www.frca.co.uk/article.aspx?articleid=228

Answer 20: D

A colloid is a suspension of particles that cannot traverse a semipermeable membrane. This suspension has a high osmolality that aids plasma expansion to an effect greater than the volume infused in patients. This temporary plasma expansion is very useful in haemorrhagic states as the colloid is initially confined to the intravascular space. Crystalloids, on the other hand, are more useful in dehydration to replace fluids in all compartments associated with electrolyte imbalances.

Further reading

Peck, T.E., Williams, M., and Hill, S.A. *Pharmacology for Anaesthesia and Intensive Care*. Cambridge: Cambridge University Press, 2003.

Answer 21: D

Diathermy is used to coagulate blood vessels and to cut or destroy tissues. It uses AC, typically at a frequency of 1 MHz, to cause the movement of ions back and forth, which results in local heating of tissue. In monopolar diathermy, current flows between an active plate with a small surface area through tissue and a neutral plate with a large area. The same amount of current flows in the two plates, but the current density is high at the active plate, resulting in cutting or coagulation. Tissue damage does not occur at the neutral plate as the current density is low. The neutral plate should be applied to dry, clean and hairless skin to allow adequate surface area to disperse the current. Furthermore, the neutral plate should not be applied on bony prominences, or over scars or metal prostheses. In bipolar diathermy, the current flows between two electrodes close to each other (e.g. as arranged at the tip of forceps). Here no neutral plate is required. Bipolar diathermy is preferred when there are concerns that use of monopolar diathermy might cause high current densities in body tissues not targeted, for example digital surgery, where current flow through the finger might be at a sufficiently high density to destroy tissues. Furthermore, bipolar diathermy is preferred in situations where pacemakers are *in situ*, as there is minimal current dispersal through other tissues, hence greatly reducing the risk of pacemaker malfunction. Cutting is achieved using a sine wave pattern of alternating current. Coagulation is achieved using a pulsed sine wave pattern of alternating current.

Further reading

Plumridge, J. Surgical diathermy. Great Ormand Street Hospital Guidelines. 2005. http://www.gosh.nhs.uk/health-professionals/clinical-guidelines/surgical-diathermy/#Rationale

Answer 22: E

Any acidic or alkaline insult to the body is initially dealt with by buffer systems. This is followed by respiratory compensation and then renal compensation which takes longer to take effect. Buffers can be intracellular or extracellular. Intracellular buffers include haemoglobin and other proteins, the phosphate buffer systems and the bicarbonate buffer system. Extracellular buffers include plasma proteins, the bicarbonate buffer system and the phosphate buffer system. When such an acidic load is injected into the body, the buffers systems will adjust themselves to minimize the decrease in pH. Action of the bicarbonate buffer system results in increased CO_2 tension in the blood which stimulates increased alveolar ventilation to expel the excess CO_2 generated – this is relatively quick. At the same time, the kidneys secrete H+ and reabsorb more bicarbonate and phosphate to buffer the H+.

Further reading

Power, I., and Kam, P. *Principles of Physiology for the Anaesthetist.* 2nd ed. London: Hodder Arnold, 2008, 253–60.

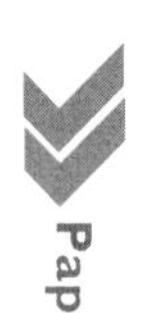

Answer 23: D

Carbon dioxide absorbers are ubiquitous in anaesthesia and allow the circle systems to be used without accumulation of CO_2. Many forms of absorbers are available, but most employ calcium hydroxide (80% of the weight of the material), which combines with CO_2 to form calcium carbonate and water. Soda lime contains small amounts of sodium hydroxide (5%) and potassium hydroxide as catalysts for the reaction. In UK preparations, the potassium hydroxide is omitted. Baralyme contains barium hydroxide (11%) as a catalyst and is not as efficient as soda lime. Silica, usually at a concentration of 1%, is added as a binding agent to create particles. 4–8 mesh size particles are selected for their optimal surface area when packed tightly. Dyes are often incorporated to show when the absorber capacity is exceeded, such as titan yellow (which changes from pink to white) and ethyl violet (which changes from white to purple) when exhausted.

Further reading

Davey, A., and Diba, A. *Ward's Anaesthetic Equipment.* 5th ed. London: Elsevier Saunders, 2005.

Answer 24: D

Oxygen reserve depends on the following:

1. FiO_2 and thus PaO_2;
2. $PaCO_2$ and alveolar ventilation – from the PaO_2 and PCO_2 relationship in the alveolus described by the alveolar gas equation; and
3. Functional residual capacity (FRC).

In this patient, increasing the respiratory rate and alveolar ventilation will decrease the $PaCO_2$, effectively creating more 'alveolar space' for oxygen. However, a larger increase in lung oxygen stores can be obtained by increasing FRC by applying positive-end expiratory pressure or by recruitment manoeuvres. Paralyzing the patient is likely to reduce the tone in the intercostal muscles and diaphragm, and thus reduce FRC.

Further reading

Yentis, S., Hirsch, N., and Smith, G. *Anaesthesia and Intensive Care A–Z.* 4th ed. London: Churchill Livingstone, 2009.

Answer 25: C

This infant has a supraventricular tachycardia (SVT) that most commonly presents as an atrioventricular re-entrant tachycardia (AVRT).

In children, an accessory atrioventricular pathway between the atria and ventricles recycles the electrical impulse back to the atria after traversing the AV node, thus causing a re-entrant tachycardia. Blocking the AV node will prevent

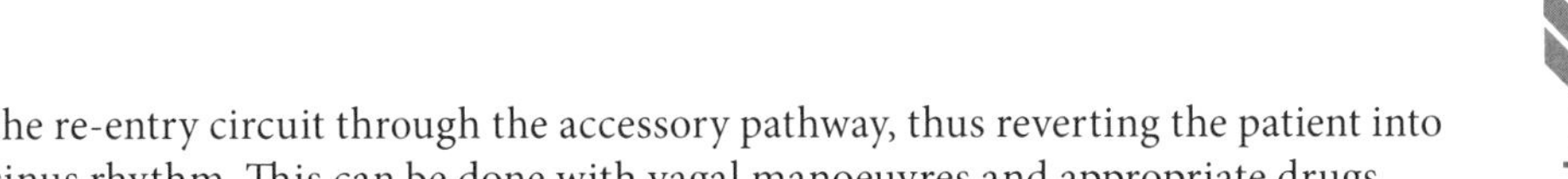

the re-entry circuit through the accessory pathway, thus reverting the patient into sinus rhythm. This can be done with vagal manoeuvres and appropriate drugs.

Applying an ice bag to the face or forehead for 5 seconds will stimulate the vagus and reduce the heart rate. The face should be covered for only 5 seconds because the infant can become apnoeic during the manoeuvre.

Gaining IV access can stress an already compromised infant; thus, vagal manoeuvres are the first choice. If IV access is *in situ*, then adenosine is equally safe and must be administered as an intravenous (IV) rapid bolus followed by 5 mL of flush to prevent plasma metabolism of adenosine from reaching its target. Although verapramil is used in adults, its side effects of bradycardia, asystole and shock could be dangerous, hence its contraindication in children. Cardiac pacing is not the appropriate management, and DC cardioversion should be reserved for the haemodynamically compromised child.

Further reading

Peck, T.E., Williams, M., and Hill, S.A. *Pharmacology for Anaesthesia and Intensive Care*. Cambridge: Cambridge University Press, 2003.

Answer 26: B

Gas cylinders used in medicine are usually made from molybdenum or chromium steel. However, aluminium cylinders are available for use within the MRI suite. Lightweight cylinders are prevalent throughout hospitals and are made from using composite materials (e.g. metal and carbon fibre). The cylinder capacity is denoted by letters. For oxygen cylinders at 137 Barr:

Size C contains 170 L;
Size D contains 340 L; and
Size E contains 680 L.

Oxygen exists in the gaseous form in cylinders, and thus the gauge pressure will allow the determination of the remaining volume of gas in the cylinder (Boyle's Law). Cylinders of nitrous oxide and carbon dioxide, however, contain a mixture of liquid and vapour. Pressure varies according to temperature (Third Perfect Gas Law), and hence if filled to maximum capacity can lead to dangerous levels of pressure. This may result in explosion of the cylinder on exposure to an increased temperature. To prevent this, cylinders are underfilled to a specified filling ratio:

Filling ratio = weight of substance contained in the cylinder / weight of water that would fill the cylinder

In the United Kingdom this ratio is 0.75, while in places with hotter climates, the ratio is lower at 0.67.

Further reading

Davey, A., and Diba, A. *Ward's Anaesthetic Equipment*. 5th ed. London: Elsevier Saunders, 2005.

Answer 27: C

The shunt in question here is due to alveolar collapse and congestion. Thus, the affected alveoli are not being ventilated despite being perfused. Increasing FiO_2 will improve the oxygen saturations but will not help to resolve the shunt. Increasing cardiac output will improve oxygen delivery to the tissues but again do little to improve the shunt in question. Laying the patient supine reduces their FRC and hence their oxygen stores. Giving the units of blood again will improve the oxygen content of blood and peripheral oxygen delivery but will not improve the shunt. The shunt can be improved in this circumstance by applying continuous positive airway pressure (CPAP). This will recruit collapsed alveoli and improve the FRC – thus more of the perfused alveoli will be ventilated and oxygenated.

Further reading

West, J.B. *Respiratory Physiology*. 7th ed. Philadelphia: Lippincott Williams and Wilkins, 2005, 55–72.

Answer 28: B

- Kernicterus can occur if bilirubin is displaced from its bond to albumin by competing drugs like sulphonamides.
- Grey baby syndrome is caused by chloramphenicol. Babies have immature glucuronidation enzymes and insufficient renal excretion, resulting in toxic chloramphenicol metabolites. This syndrome has the predominantly cardiovascular effects of hypotension, cyanosis and ultimately cardiovascular collapse.
- Tetracyclines cause tooth enamel dysplasia and bone growth inhibition.
- Ototoxicity is caused by streptomycin.
- Neural tube defects are due to valproic acid.

Further reading

Peck, T.E., Williams, M., and Hill, S.A. *Pharmacology for Anaesthesia and Intensive Care*. Cambridge: Cambridge University Press, 2003.

Answer 29: D

The rotameter is a variable-orifice constant-pressure flow meter. The flow meter consists of a tapered tube (narrow at the bottom) that houses a bobbin. This bobbin is supported by a column of gas introduced via a needle valve controlled by a dial. As the gas flow increases, the upward pressure on the bobbin increases. This results in the bobbin rising and the annular orifice around it increasing. The increase in the annular area reduces the pressure. The bobbin continues to rise until the pressure generated by the driving gas matches the force of gravity acting on the bobbin. Thus, a constant pressure is maintained across the bobbin. The system requires calibration for each gas, and readings are taken from the top of the

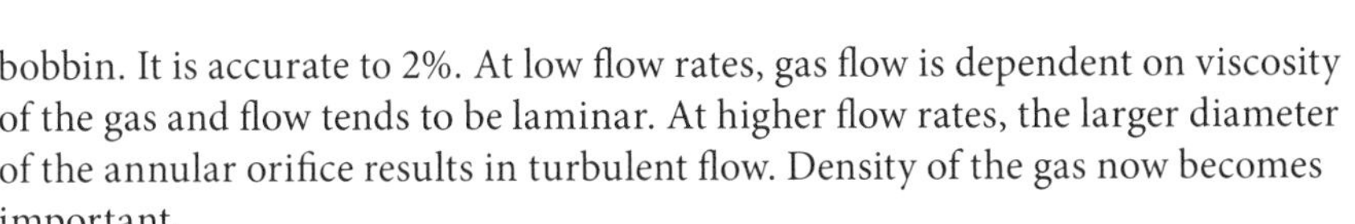

bobbin. It is accurate to 2%. At low flow rates, gas flow is dependent on viscosity of the gas and flow tends to be laminar. At higher flow rates, the larger diameter of the annular orifice results in turbulent flow. Density of the gas now becomes important.

Further reading

Davies, P., and Kenny, G. *Basic Physics and Measurement in Anaesthesia*. 5th ed. London: Butterworth Heinemann, 2005.

Answer 30: A

This child will need nebulized salbutamol. Her condition is stable with an SpO_2 of 95% on air with no accessory muscle use. Thus, oxygen is not necessary. Cromolyn sodium, a mast cell stabilizer and anti-inflammatory drug, is useful in asthma prophylaxis and will not help in this acute situation. Both IV steroids and subcutaneous adrenaline are reserved for severe asthmatics.

Further reading

Peck, T.E., Williams, M., and Hill, S.A. *Pharmacology for Anaesthesia and Intensive Care*. Cambridge: Cambridge University Press, 2003.

PAPER 5 QUESTIONS

Question 1

A fit and well 37-weeks-pregnant mother attends an anaesthetic antenatal clinic for assessment, prior to her elective Caesarean section. Routine blood tests show a haemoglobin of 10.0 g/dl with a mean corpuscular volume (MCV) of 89, platelets of 160 and white blood cell count (WCC) of 14. These findings are most consistent with which of the following?

A. Iron deficiency anaemia
B. Dilutional anaemia of pregnancy
C. Myelodysplasia
D. Folic acid deficiency
E. Pancytopaenia

Question 2

Low-molecular-weight heparin (LMWH) therapy was initiated ante-natally on a 28-year-old woman on long-term anticoagulation with warfarin. She is day 1 post-delivery, and the obstetricians feel she is at increased risk of perineal haematoma. Which of the following would be the best post-natal anticoagulation strategy?

A. Intravenous heparin infusion with close monitoring of activated partial thromboplastin time (APTT).
B. Warfarin for 5 days, and then switch over to LMWH.
C. Start fondaparinux.
D. Intravenous heparin infusion for 5 days, followed by fondaparinux.
E. LMWH for 7 days, and then switch over to warfarin.

Question 3

Which of the following statements regarding the Proseal™ laryngeal mask airway (LMA) is most accurate?

A. It is a single-use device.
B. It is not suitable in the paediatric population.
C. It allows positive pressure ventilation up to 30 cm of water.
D. It is difficult to site a gastric tube when the Proseal is used.
E. It has been proved to prevent aspiration.

Question 4

A 35-year-old female is pre-operatively assessed to have a hysteroscopy. Her body mass index (BMI) is 38. Which of the following statements best describes her BMI?

A. Super-morbidly obese
B. Morbidly obese
C. Normal BMI
D. Overweight
E. Obese

Question 5

A 35-year-old pregnant patient is scheduled for an elective lower section Caesarean section (LSCS) due to a previous LSCS. She is 37 weeks pregnant and is HIV-positive. Her viral load is 436, and her CD4 count is 100. She was started on an infusion of zidovudine before LSCS. Which of the following statements regarding this scenario is most correct?

A. Zidovudine will protect the mother from peri-operative infections.
B. The drug azidothymidine (AZT) would have been a better choice in this scenario.
C. Paracetamol is very safe as an analgesic.
D. Thymidine kinase is essential for zidovudine to act.
E. Zidovudine will have a partial effect on human DNA.

Question 6

Which of the following regarding giving sets and filters used for fluid administration is false?

A. Most giving sets utilize depth filters.
B. Screen filters increase in efficiency with each unit of blood filtered.
C. Platelets should be administered via a giving set not previously used for blood.
D. Blood should be given through a filter with a pore size of 170–200 μm.
E. Epidural filters have a pore size of 0.2 μm.

Question 7

A 19-year-old man is involved in a road traffic accident and is brought in with haemorrhagic shock. He undergoes an explorative laparotomy during which you notice his blood sugar level to be rising. He is not known to have diabetes, and a recent glucose tolerance test, during a private health check-up, was entirely normal. Which of the following reasons is most likely to be the cause of the hyperglycaemia?

A. Lactate acid in Hartmann's solution
B. Catecholamines and cortisol released as part of the stress response to trauma and surgery
C. A new diagnosis of diabetes
D. Increased thyroid hormone production as part of the stress response
E. Increased gluconeogenesis and glycogenolysis, and a decrease in insulin secretion and activity

Question 8

A 45-year-old man has been recently diagnosed with diabetes mellitus. The endocrinologist wants to start a drug from the sulphonyurea group. Which of the following statements best describes the mechanism of action of sulphonyurea drugs?

A. They displace insulin from B-cells in the islets of Langerhans.
B. They delay uptake of glucose from the gut.
C. They inhibit hepatic and renal gluconeogenesis.
D. They are competitive inhibitors of alpha-glucosidase.
E. They enhance tyrosine kinase activity within the insulin receptor.

Question 9

Regarding the ultrasound probe used in medicine, which of the following statements is incorrect?

A. A frequency of 10 MHz is used to visualize blood vessels in the neck.
B. Piezoelectric crystals are used to detect the signal.
C. Ultrasound waves are partially reflected back at tissue interfaces.
D. Resolution is increased at higher frequency.
E. Penetration is reduced at higher frequency.

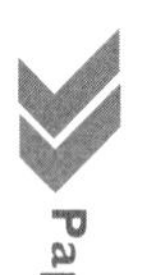

Question 10

A 45-year-old man is reviewed in a pain clinic. He suffers from trigeminal neuralgia. On examination of his maxillary area, he describes stabbing pain in response to normal touch. Which of the following statements best describes what he is experiencing?

A. Neuropathic pain
B. Primary hyperalgesia
C. Allodynia
D. Spinal cord wind-up
E. Neuralgia

Question 11

Which of the following statements is most correct regarding peri-operative steroid supplementation in patients already on steroid therapy?

A. Patients taking 5 mg prednisolone daily do not have a normal hypothalamic–pituitary axis (HPA).
B. Patients taking 15 mg prednisolone daily do not need peri-operative supplementation.
C. 25 mg hydrocortisone at induction covers the requirements for minor surgery.
D. Moderate surgery requires a further 200 mg hydrocortisone to be administered in the first 24 hours of the post-operative period.
E. The HPA is not supressed with long-term steroids.

Question 12

The Oxylog 3000 portable ventilator is frequently used to ventilate intubated patients who are being transferred. Which of the following statements is false?

A. It is driven by a high-pressure gas source.
B. It can be used in either the volume- or pressure-controlled mode.
C. It has a gas consumption of up to 1 L/min for internal control.
D. It is suitable for use in a 4-year-old patient.
E. It cannot be used for non-invasive ventilation.

Question 13

You are called to review a patient with anorexia nervosa in accident and emergency resuscitation (A&E resus) who has taken a thyroxine overdose in an attempt to increase her basal metabolic rate. Which of the following statements best defines basal metabolic rate?

A. Rate of metabolism at rest in an individual in a thermoneutral environment
B. Rate of heat production in an individual who is at mental and physical rest, in a thermoneutral environment, 12–14 hours after a meal
C. An average of an individual's metabolic rates measured at 3-hour intervals during a 24-hour period and during all types of activity
D. Rate of energy production in an individual at rest
E. Rate of heat production in an individual who is at physical rest in a thermoneutral environment 24 hours after a meal

Question 14

A pharmaceutical representative describes a drug used to treat hyperthyroidism. This drug is a prodrug that prevents the synthesis of new T3 and T4 by inhibiting the oxidation of iodide to iodine and by inhibiting thyroid peroxidase. This drug does not break down stored T3 and T4; hence, the patient will have to be on this drug for some weeks before a euthyroid state is achieved. Which is the drug being described?

A. Thyroxine
B. Propylthiouracil
C. Carbimazole
D. Iodides
E. Propranolol

Question 15

Oxygen is stored in vacuum-insulated evaporators (VIEs). Choose one statement from the following list which is most accurate.

A. Refrigeration is a mandatory component of the VIE.
B. Oxygen passes through a superheater prior to pipeline entry.
C. A safety valve maintains the pressure in the VIE at 134 bar.
D. Liquid oxygen is stored at –130°C within the chamber.
E. Liquid oxygen enters the pipeline.

Question 16

A child playing in the garden trips and falls. He sustains a bruise over his left knee. The child's pain is alleviated as his mother rubs the area with her hand. This phenomenon is best explained by which of the following?

A. The gate control theory of pain and closure of the 'gate' from A beta fibre stimulation
B. The gate control theory of pain and opening of the 'gate' from A beta fibre stimulation
C. Stimulation of c-fibres and closure of the 'gate' in the subtantia gelatinosa
D. Stimulation of A delta fibres peripherally
E. Production of histamine locally and inhibition of peripheral pain transmission

Question 17

Which of the following statement is most true of acetazolamide?

A. Increases carbonic anhydrase synthesis
B. Is a strong diuretic
C. Causes a metabolic acidosis
D. Produces hypokalaemic hypochloraemic alkalosis
E. Enhances hydrogen ion excretion by the kidneys

Question 18

All of the following are safety features of modern anaesthetic machines except:

A. An emergency oxygen flush provides flow rates in excess of 35 L/min.
B. Oxygen is fed downstream of other gases.
C. Piped gases are connected to Schrader sockets on the anaesthetic machine.
D. A pressure-relieving valve is set at 30 kPa to prevent damage to the machine.
E. An oxygen failure device will trigger if the oxygen pressure drops below 200 kPa.

Question 19

A 35-year-old patient with acute liver failure develops a metabolic acidosis. Respiratory compensation is triggered by which one of the following mechanisms specifically?

A. Aortic and carotid body chemoreceptor stimulation with afferent nerves travelling via the glossopharyngeal and vagus nerves, respectively, and the central medullay chemoreceptors
B. Aortic and carotid body chemoreceptor stimulation with afferent nerves travelling via the glossopharyngeal and vagus nerves, respectively
C. Aortic and carotid body chemoreceptor stimulation with afferent impulses travelling in the vagus and glossopharyngeal nerves, respectively
D. Aortic and carotid body chemoreceptors travelling via the vagus and glossophryngeal nerves, respectively, and the central medullary chemoreceptors
E. Central chemoreceptors in the respiratory centre of the medulla only

Question 20

Some of ethanol's properties are described below. Which of the following would be the most untrue statement regarding ethanol?

A. Alcoholism results from ethanol.
B. Methanol poisoning is treated with ethanol.
C. Ethanol is an anaesthetic and tocolytic agent.
D. Ethanol is metabolized to acetaldehyde via the tricarboxylic acid (TCA) cycle.
E. At high concentrations, ethanol follows first-order kinetics.

Question 21

The Bernoulli effect is used in all but which of the following equipment?

A. Gas-driven nebulizer
B. Ultrasonic nebulizer
C. Venturi mask
D. Suction equipment
E. Scavenging equipment

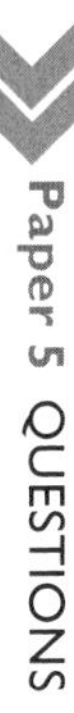

Question 22

2 L of 5% dextrose is given intravenously to a fit and healthy medical student at rest over half an hour. The diuresis which ensues promptly is most likely to be due to which of the following?

A. Increased renin secretion
B. Decreased anti-diuretic hormone release
C. Increased anti-diuretic hormone release
D. Decreased aldosterone release
E. Increased vasopressin levels

Question 23

Which of the anti-emetics below is correctly matched with its receptor?

A. Dopamine antagonists: cannabinoids
B. Anticholinergics: hyoscine
C. 5HT3 antagonists: promethazine
D. Antihistaminic: chlorpromazine
E. NK1 receptor antagonist: amitryptalline

Question 24

Which of the following statements regarding the safety classification of medical equipment is true?

A. Nerve stimulators for assessing neuromuscular blockade are Class II equipment.
B. Fuses are not required for Class I equipment.
C. Type B equipment allows a maximal leakage of 0.05 amps.
D. Class II equipment is earthed.
E. Class III equipment incorporates internal power sources.

Question 25

A 29-year-old pregnant woman with sickle cell trait attends a conference at a high altitude in Peru. She develops a urine infection and becomes hypothermic at 35.6°C. Which of the following factors would tend to decrease the release of oxygen from haemoglobin?

A. Pregnancy
B. Altitude
C. Sickle cell trait
D. Decreased body temperature
E. Metabolic acidosis from urosepsis

Question 26

A 7-year-old boy, previously fit, is in the recovery bay after an appendectomy. He is now complaining of severe pain that is sharp and localized to the surgical site. He is awake and haemodynamically stable. His analgesic regime thus far has been intravenous (IV) fentanyl intraoperatively 50 mcg, surgical infiltration of 0.25% bupivacaine (15 mL), 25 mg of rectal diclofenac and 300 mg IV paracetamol. What would be the most appropriate analgesic option for him in recovery now?

A. Codeine phosphate 20 mg orally
B. Codeine phosphate 20 mg intramuscularly (IM)
C. Morphine 0.1 mg/kg intravenous bolus
D. An intravenous morphine infusion at 10 mcg/kg/hour
E. IM morphine 2 mg in recovery

Question 27

A patient has suffered ventricular fibrillation secondary to an electric shock. Which of the following is likely to have been the cause?

A. A high-voltage direct current (DC) shock
B. A 150 mA current applied across the torso
C. A current of 5 mA applied to the hand
D. A current of 3 μA applied to a saline drip administered via the internal jugular vein
E. A current of 50 mA applied directly to the sternum

Question 28

A patient on the intensive care unit with a massive subarachnid haemorrhage is to undergo brain stem testing to establish brain stem death, prior to referral to the organ retrieval team. All but which of the following cranial nerve pathways are tested?

A. Afferent cranial nerve II
B. Afferent cranial nerve X
C. Efferent cranial nerve VII
D. Afferent cranial nerve V
E. Efferent cranial nerve XII

Question 29

A 45-year-old male admitted in hospital with pneumonia complains of palpitations. His blood pressure is 100/60 mm Hg with a regular heart rate of 160 beats per minute. The palpitations are not associated with chest pain. A 12 lead electrocardiogram (ECG) shows the duration of the QRS complex to be 0.10 s. Which of the following immediate treatments is most appropriate for this patient?

A. Amiodarone 300 mg
B. Digoxin 0.5 mg
C. Adenosine 6 mg
D. Esmolol 100 mg
E. DC cardioversion

Question 30

Which of the following statements is most accurate regarding the depth of anaesthesia monitoring?

A. The PRST (pressure, rate, sweating and tears) scoring system is most reliable.
B. Auditory evoked potentials are more sensitive than somatosensory evoked potentials.
C. A bispectral index of 80 correlates with general anaesthesia.
D. Entropy increases with increasing depth of anaesthesia.
E. Nerve stimulators are the mainstay of monitoring.

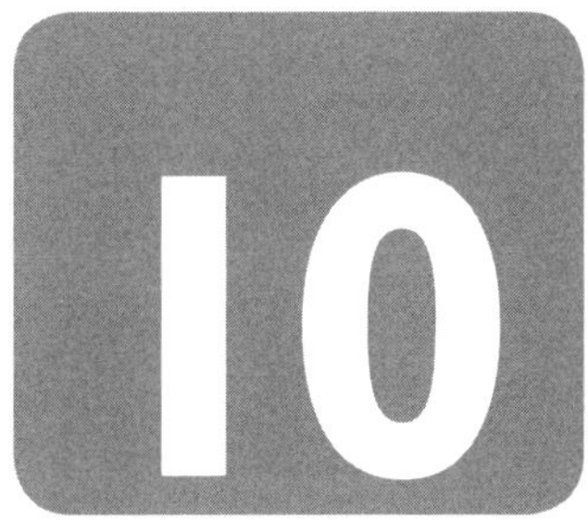

PAPER 5 ANSWERS

Answer 1: B

Anaemia in pregnancy can have multiple aetiologies. With a normal mean corpuscular volume (MCV), the most likely cause is dilutional anaemia of pregnancy. Anaemia of pregnancy arises as a result of the disproportionate increase in plasma relative to haemoglobin, resulting in dilution of the haemoglobin concentration. A low MVC would be observed with iron deficiency anaemia, and a high MVC with B_{12}–folate deficiency. A mixed picture of iron and B_{12}–folate deficiency could result in the case given here, but this is unlikely. Pancytopaenia is defined as low haemoglobin (Hb), low white blood cell count (WCC) and low platelets – which this woman does not have. Myelodysplasia is unlikely to manifest as solely a reduced Hb and is more likely to be seen with high/low WCC and/or high/low platelets.

Further reading

Spoors, C., and Kiff, K. *Training in Anaesthesia: The Essential Curriculum*. Oxford: Oxford University Press, 2010, 468.

Answer 2: E

Low-molecular-weight heparin (LMWH) is appropriate for postpartum thromboprophylaxis, although if women are receiving long-term anticoagulation with warfarin, this can be restarted when the risk of haemorrhage is low, usually 5–7 days after delivery.

Both warfarin and LMWH are safe when breastfeeding.

Warfarin can be safely used following delivery and in breastfeeding mothers, although it requires close monitoring and visits to an anticoagulant clinic. It carries an increased risk of postpartum haemorrhage and perineal haematoma compared with LMWH. It is not appropriate for those women requiring 7 days of postpartum prophylaxis.

It is unknown whether fondaparinux is excreted in breast milk, and although oral absorption seems unlikely, it should be avoided in this setting.

Further reading

Royal College of Obstetricians. *Green Top Guideline 37*. November. London: Royal College of Obstetricians, 2009.

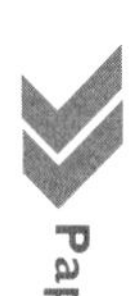

Answer 3: C

The Proseal™ laryngeal mask airway (LMA) is a modified LMA and houses a second lumen which ends at the distal tip. This port sits over the entry to the oesophagus when the device is correctly sited and allows the passage of an orogastric tube. Furthermore, this lumen may afford a route for the drainage of regurgitated fluid. However, it cannot prevent aspiration, particular if the patient vomits. The cuff provides a 'high-integrity seal', and positive pressure ventilation up to 30 cm of water can be achieved. The presence of the oesophageal port will also minimize gastric insufflation, and postoperative nausea and vomiting are reported to be reduced. The device is manufactured in many sizes, including a size 1 which is recommended for neonates.

Further reading

Davey, A., and Diba, A. *Ward's Anaesthetic Equipment.* 5th ed. London: Elsevier Saunders, 2005.
LMA North America. http://www.lmana.com

Answer 4: E

Body mass index (BMI) is described as a ratio of an individual's weight in kg and their height in metres squared:

$$\text{BMI} = \text{weight} / (\text{height [M]} \times \text{height [M]})$$

Ranges are as follows:

- Underweight: <18.49
- Normal: 18.5–24.99
- Overweight: 25–29.99
- Obese class I: 30–34.99
- Obese class II: 35–39.99
- Obese class III: >40

Further reading

World Health Organization. Global database on body mass index. http://apps.who.int/bmi/index.jsp?introPage = intro_3.html

Answer 5: D

Zidovudine is AZT (azidothymidine, or 3-azido-3-deoxythymidine) and has been started to protect the baby from vertical transmission. AZT's toxicity is enhanced by co-administration of enzyme inhibitor drugs like paracetamol, cimetidine and probenecid due to decreased glucoronidation.

AZT works as an antiviral by inhibiting the synthesis of DNA within the virus. AZT is converted to the relevant nucleotide that has antiviral activity.

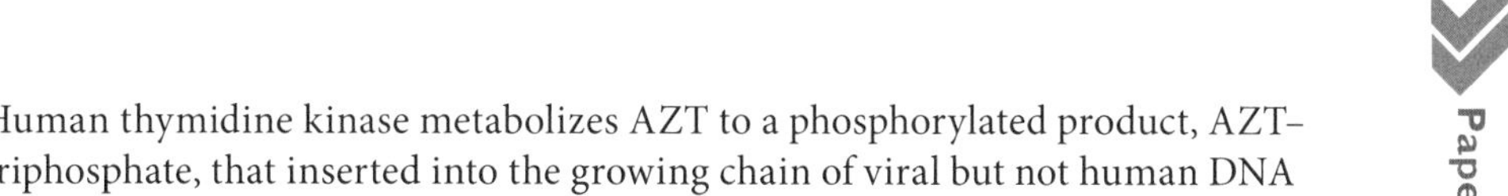

Human thymidine kinase metabolizes AZT to a phosphorylated product, AZT-triphosphate, that inserted into the growing chain of viral but not human DNA by reverse transcriptase. Because AZT lacks a hydroxyl group at the 3′ position, another 5′-3′ phosphodiester linkage cannot be formed. The virus cannot replicate as the DNA chain synthesis is halted.

Further reading

Peck, T.E., Williams, M., and Hill, S.A. *Pharmacology for Anaesthesia and Intensive Care*. Cambridge: Cambridge University Press, 2003.

Answer 6: A

All fluids administered intravenously (IV) must be filtered to prevent exposing the patient to microemboli. Microaggregates frequently form in stored blood products and may cause significant pulmonary emboli if not removed. Typically, most filters are of the screen type and act as molecular sieves. Screen filters for blood products typically have pore sizes of 170 to 200 micrometres (aka microns or μm). The efficiency of these filters increases with each unit of blood, as the pore size decreases with use. Platelets should not be administered via a giving set previously used to deliver blood as they can be adsorbed onto erythrocytes captured on the filter. Depth filters, composed of packed synthetic material, absorb unwanted particles down to a size of 10 μm. Epidural filters have pore sizes typically in the region of 0.2 μm to filter out bacterial contaminants.

Further reading

Association of Anaesthetists of Great Britain and Ireland. Blood transfusion and the anaesthetist and management of massive haemorrhage: AAGBI safety guideline. 2010. http://www.aagbi.org/sites/default/files/massive_haemorrhage_2010_0.pdf

Davey, A., and Diba, A. *Ward's Anaesthetic Equipment*. 5th ed. London: Elsevier Saunders, 2005.

Tyagi, A., Kumar, R., Bhattacharya, A., and Sethi, A.K. Filters in anaesthesia and intensive care. *Anaesth Intensive Care* (2003) 31(4): 418–33.

Answer 7: E

This patient is exhibiting one of the many physiological responses to surgery and trauma. Surgery and trauma evoke a catabolic response as the body attempts to compensate for the insult and initiate healing. The response has some aspects which are beneficial and others which are potentially harmful. Indeed, part of peri-operative care is to minimize the negative aspects of the surgical stress response.

Surgery or trauma results in the activation of the sympathetic system and the release of pituitary hormones. Blood glucose levels increase as a result of the following:

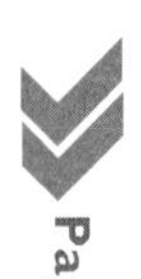

1. Decreased insulin secretion – alpha adrenergic effect;
2. Increased growth hormone secretion – this inhibits glucose uptake; and
3. Increased gluconeogenesis (and possibly glycogenolysis) mediated by cortisol and circulating catecholamines.

For details of the remaining effects of the stress response to surgery, see the reference given here.

Further reading

Spoors, C., and Kiff, K. *Training in Anaesthesia: The Essential Curriculum*. Oxford: Oxford University Press, 2010, 466.

Answer 8: A

Sulphonylureas bind to the ATP K+ channel on the B-cell membrane and depolarize the cell to secrete insulin. Hence, in insulin-dependent diabetes mellitus (IDDM) patients who have nonfunctioning B-cells, they are not very useful. Sulphonylureas also reduce glucose by inhibiting liver production of glucose and reducing peripheral resistance to insulin.

The biguanides inhibit hepatic and renal gluconeogenesis and, along with acarbose, inhibit uptake of glucose from the gut.

Further reading

Peck, T.E., Williams, M., and Hill, S.A. *Pharmacology for Anaesthesia and Intensive Care*. Cambridge: Cambridge University Press, 2003.

Answer 9: A

The frequency of ultrasound is in excess of 20 KHz. The frequency used for medical imaging is in the range of 1–20 MHz. The ultrasound is generated by distorting piezoelectric crystals using a rapidly changing electric field. Some of the incident waves are reflected at the interface of tissues with different densities. These reflected waves are detected by the crystals and transduced into electrical signals, which are then used to generate an image. High-frequency waves generate higher resolution, but have low penetration as the high-frequency sound waves are readily absorbed by tissues. Conversely, low-frequency waves have better penetration but poorer resolution. The time taken to detect a reflected wave is indicative of the depth of the reflecting structure, while the amount of reflection gives information on the density differences at the tissue.

Further reading

Anaesthesia UK. Ultrasound. http://www.frca.co.uk/SectionContents.aspx?sectionid=86

Answer 10: C

This man is experiencing neuropathic pain (i.e. pain from injury to or as a result of the dysfunction of neuronal tissue). More specifically, his symptoms can be catagorized as allodynia, which is described as a painful sensation in response to a normal non-noxious stimulus. Hyperalgesia is defined as an increased response to a normally noxious stimulus (primary – referring to that part of the hyperalgesia occurring in the area of innervation of the injured nerve; and secondary – referring to hyperalgesia in the area surrounding that of the injured nerve). Neuralgia describes pain from the distribution of a particular nerve or nerves, as with trigeminal neuralgia. Spinal cord wind-up refers to a phenomenon whereby noxious input into the spinal cord results in increased excitability of neurons in the spinal cord – the phenomenon is 'frequency dependent' and pertains to C-fibre input.

Further reading

Clifton, B., Armstrong S., et al. *Primary FRCA in a Box.* London: Royal Society of Medicine Press Ltd, 2007, 224–6.

World Health Organization. Global database on Body Mass Index. http://apps.who.int/bmi/index.jsp?introPage = intro_3.html

Answer 11: C

Peri-operative steroid supplementation will depend on the patient's pre-operative steroid dose and type of surgery.

Patients on <10 mg prednisolone daily have a normal hypothalamic–pituitary axis (HPA) and thus do not need supplementation.

Patients on >10 mg prednisolone daily will need peri-operative steroid cover as follows:

- Minor surgery: IV hydrocortisone 25 mg at induction only.
- Moderate surgery: IV hydrocortisone 25 mg on induction + 100 mg hydrocortisone over 24 hours post-operatively.
- Major surgery: IV hydrocortisone 25 mg on induction + 100 mg hydrocortisone per day for 72 hours post-operatively.
- Long-term steroids would suppress the HPA.

Further reading

Peck, T.E., Williams, M., and Hill, S.A. *Pharmacology for Anaesthesia and Intensive Care.* Cambridge: Cambridge University Press, 2003.

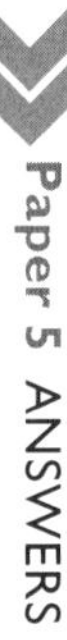

Answer 12: E

The Oxylog 3000 is a portable ventilator that houses a microprocessor which allows sophisticated ventilation modes. It is capable of delivering tidal volumes in the range of 50 to 2000 mL and thus can be used in the paediatric patient. The Oxylog 3000 is driven by a high-pressure oxygen source, and it is possible to adjust the delivered oxygen concentration. It has a variety of ventilatory modes including intermittent positive pressure ventilation, mandatory ventilation and pressure support. Furthermore, it can be used to provide non-invasive ventilation and continuous positive airway pressure. It is important to note that the Oxylog 3000 consumes gas (up to 1 L/min) for operations other than delivering tidal volumes. A rechargeable battery is incorporated to power the electrical components required for operating the microprocessor and display panels.

Further reading

Dräger Medical. Oxylog 3000. Technical data sheet. http://www.ivermedi.com/attachments/pdf/oxylog_3000.pdf

Fludger, S., and Klein, A. Portable ventilators. *Contin Educ Anaesth Crit Care Pain* (2008) 8 (6): 199–203.

Answer 13: B

Metabolic rate is defined as the rate of energy liberation per unit time:

Energy liberation = work done externally + energy stored + heat energy released

Basal metabolic rate is defined as the rate at which metabolism occurs or energy is liberated per unit time when an individual is at rest (i.e. not doing any work) in a thermoneutral (comfortable) environment (minimal energy expenditure to maintain body temperature), 12–14 hours since their last meal (energy from food has been largely if not completely stored). At this stage, energy liberation equals heat energy released.

Factors affecting metabolic rate include recent intake of food, age, sex, lactation, emotions, circulating thyroid hormone levels, muscular activity and ambient temperatures.

Further reading

Ganong, W.F. *Review of Medical Physiology*. 22nd ed. New York: McGraw-Hill, 2005, 279–82.

Answer 14: C

Carbimazole, an anti-thyroid agent, is converted to its active form after absorption. It inhibits the enzyme thyroid peroxidase that is needed for synthesis of thyroid hormones. As it acts by inhibiting thyroid hormone synthesis and not by breaking

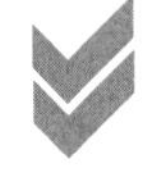

down preformed T3 and T4, the patient will benefit from this therapy only after some weeks after depletion of stores. Propylthiouracil prevents tyrosine iodination and peripheral conversion of T4 to T3.

Propranolol is a therapeutic adjuvant in thyrotoxicosis. It blocks peripheral conversion of T4 to T3 and counteracts the sympathetic stimulation.

Lugol's iodine and potassium iodide inhibit the formation and release of thyroid hormones. Onset of action is approximately 72 hours. They also reduce the size and vascularity of the thyroid gland, and hence are used before resecting a hyperplastic thyroid gland.

Further reading

Peck, T.E., Williams, M., and Hill, S.A. *Pharmacology for Anaesthesia and Intensive Care*. Cambridge: Cambridge University Press, 2003.

Answer 15: B

In most hospitals, liquid oxygen is stored at –160 to –180°C within a vacuum-insulated container. At this temperature, the saturated vapour pressure of oxygen is 7 bar. If the temperature increases, a safety valve opens to vent gas so as to maintain safe pressures. Venting of gas allows more evaporation of liquid oxygen which reduces the temperature (latent heat of evaporation). This, together with the efficient vacuum insulation, obviates the need for refrigeration. Oxygen gas is drawn from the top of the assembly and warmed by passing through a super heater, prior to entry into the pipeline. This allows warming the oxygen to ambient temperature. Furthermore, a pressure-reducing valve ensures that a pipeline pressure of 4.1 bar is achieved.

Further reading

Davies, P., and Kenny, G. *Basic Physics and Measurement in Anaesthesia*. 5th ed. London: Butterworth Heinemann, 2005.

Answer 16: A

The gate control theory of pain was proposed by Melzack and Wall in 1965. The theory proposes that pain pathways travel through a 'gate' located in the substantia gelatinosa in the spinal cord en route to the brain. It follows that the transmission of pain can be modulated at this site. The gate can be closed by input from larger-diameter ascending fibres (A-beta fibres) and descending fibres, and opened by small-diameter C-fibres. A delta fibres (pin prick and temperature sensation) open the gate by inhibiting an inhibitory interneuron but also close the gate as they activate descending inhibitory pathways as they project cranially. Thus this woman is stimulating adjacently lying A-beta fibres by rubbing, which serve to close the gate.

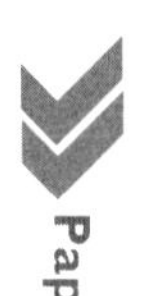

Further reading

Clifton, B., Armstrong S., et al. *Primary FRCA in a Box*. London: Royal Society of Medicine Press Ltd, 2007, 225.

Yentis, S., Hirsch, N., and Smith, G. *Anaesthesia and Intensive Care A–Z*. 4th ed. London: Churchill Livingstone, 2009.

Answer 17: C

Acetazolamide is used as prophylaxis in acute mountain sickness. The drug needs to be started a few days before reaching higher altitudes. Its dosage varies from 125 mg to 1000 mg per day depending on the ascent from sea level.

The normal physiological response at high altitude (low oxygen levels) is hyperventilation. This leads to reduced carbon dioxide (acid) *in vivo* and metabolic alkalosis. To correct this metabolic alkalosis, the kidney excessively excretes bicarbonate, but it takes a few days to normalize the alkalosis. Acetazolamide accelerates this process of excessive bicarbonate loss from the kidneys, thereby creating an acidosis. Acidifying the blood stimulates ventilation, thus increasing the amount of oxygen in the blood.

Thus, acetazolamide speeds up the acclimatization process at high altitudes to reduce symptoms. In serious mountain sickness, descent to a lower elevation is advised.

Further reading

Peck, T.E., Williams, M., and Hill, S.A. *Pharmacology for Anaesthesia and Intensive Care*. Cambridge: Cambridge University Press, 2003.

Answer 18: C

The modern anaesthetic machine has numerous safety features. The most important is the oxygen failure device, which must not be electronic. British Standard BS4272 states that this fail-safe should trigger when the pressure drops below 200 kPa and should be powered by oxygen pressure alone. The risk of delivering hypoxic mixtures is minimized by the addition of downstream oxygen to all other gases. Furthermore, the oxygen and nitrous oxide flow controls are interlinked, and it is not possible to deliver less than 25% oxygen when nitrous oxide is used. In an emergency, the oxygen flush will deliver 35 to 70 L/min. Damage to the vaporizer and rotameters by untoward high pressure is avoided by a pressure-releasing valve situated on the back bar, which will vent if the pressure exceeds 30 to 40 kPa. Flexible hoses connecting piped gases to the anaesthetic machine are colour coded, and they have Schrader sockets at the wall and a non-interchangeable screw thread system at the anaesthetic machine.

Further reading

Sinclair, C.M., Thadsad, M.K., and Barker, I. Modern anaesthetic machines. *Contin Educ Anaesth Crit Care Pain* (2006) 6 (2): 75–78.

Answer 19: D

Breathing is controlled by many mechanisms, including chemoreceptors. Chemoreceptors are located peripherally in the aortic arch and carotid bodies, with their afferents passing via the vagus and glossopharyngeal nerves, respectively. These are stimulated by a drop in PaO_2, a rise in $PaCO_2$ and a rise in hydrogen ion concentration. Stimulation results in the increase of alveolar ventilation. Central medullary chemoreceptors are exposed to hydrogen ions in the cerebrospinal fluid (CSF), and a rise in this will cause an increase in alveolar ventilation. The increase in alveolar ventilation brought about by a metabolic acidosis results in enhanced excretion of carbon dioxide, and thus reduces H+ concentration in blood. This relatively short-term compensatory mechanism provides a bridge for establishing a more sustainable renal compensation.

Further reading

Yentis, S., Hirsch, N., and Smith, G. *Anaesthesia and Intensive Care A–Z*. 4th ed. London: Churchill Livingstone, 2009.

Answer 20: E

Ethanol, commonly referred to as alcohol, is widely drunk throughout the world. It has been used in medicine as an anaesthetic and tocolytic agent. Ethanol can be used to treat methanol poisoning as well as chronic pain (as an injectate to destroy neural tissue). The tricarboxylic acid (TCA) cycle metabolizes ethanol to acetaldehyde with the help of the enzyme alcohol dehydrogenase. This enzyme is produced by the liver and is limited; hence, at low concentrations ethanol follows first-order kinetics but switches over to zero-order kinetics at higher ethanol concentrations.

Further reading

Peck, T.E., Williams, M., and Hill, S.A. *Pharmacology for Anaesthesia and Intensive Care*. Cambridge: Cambridge University Press, 2003.

Answer 21: B

Fluid flowing through a constriction gains kinetic energy and hence accelerates. To maintain a constant net energy within the system, the potential energy drops. This results in a reduced pressure distal to the constriction and is known as the Bernoulli Effect. The pressure drop may be of sufficient magnitude to entrain fluid or gas from a port just distal to the constriction. This is the Venturi Principle and is exploited in a variety of devices including suction apparatus, scavenging equipment and Venturi valves. The entrainment ratio is the entrainment flow in relation to the driving flow. The amount of entrainment is determined by the dimensions of the constrictions and the viscosity, density and flow rate of the driving gas. In the gas driven nebulizer, gas flowing through a constriction creates enough negative pressure to nebulize water from a nearby source. The ultrasonic nebulizer, on the other hand, uses a vibrating surface to generate water droplets.

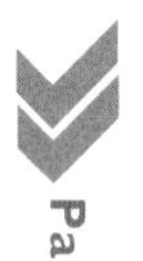

Further reading

Yentis, S., Hirsch, N., and Smith, G. *Anaesthesia and Intensive Care A–Z*. 4th ed. London: Churchill Livingstone, 2009.

Answer 22: B

Administration of 2 L of 5% dextrose IV to an individual is analogous to giving a 2 L water infusion as the dextrose is immediately metabolized. This will result in the following:

1. Decreased blood osmolality – stimulating hypothalamic osmoreceptors and decreasing the release of anti-diuretic hormone;
2. Suppression of thirst;
3. Increased renal blood flow and thus glomerular filtration rate (GFR); and
4. Hyponatraemia and direct stimulation of aldosterone release.

Vasopressin is an alternative name for anti-diuretic hormone, and it decreases secretion of renin. The regulation of intravascular volume and osmolality is complex and interlinked. The references given here explain the mechanisms involved.

Further reading

Lote, C.J. *Principles of Renal Physiology*. 4th ed. Dordrecht, the Netherlands: Kluwer Academic, 2000, 96–107.
Yentis, S., Hirsch, N., and Smith, G. *Anaesthesia and Intensive Care A–Z*. 4th ed. London: Churchill Livingstone, 2009.

Answer 23: B

- *Dopamine antagonists*: chlorpromazine, prochlorperazine, droperidol, domperidone and metoclopramide.
- *Anticholinergics*: hyoscine, atropine and glycopyrrolate.
- *5HT3 antagonists*: ondansetron, tropisetron and granisetron.
- *Antihistaminics*: cyclizine and promethazine.
- *Amitriptyline* is not an anti-emetic. Steroids (dexamethasone), acupuncture (P6 point) and cannabinoids have anti-emetic properties.
- *NK1 receptor antagonists* are used as anti-emetics in cancer chemotherapy such as aprepitant.

Further reading

Peck, T.E., Williams, M., and Hill, S.A. *Pharmacology for Anaesthesia and Intensive Care*. Cambridge: Cambridge University Press, 2003.

Answer 24: F

Electronic equipment needs to meet safety standards as set out in the British Standard EN 60601 document 'Safety of medical electrical equipment'. This document requires all electrical equipment to be categorized into one of three classes:

- Class I: any conductive part of such equipment which may contact the user are earthed (i.e. grounded). A fuse is incorporated such that the fuse disintegrates if the user becomes part of the circuit.
- Class II: The user is protected from making contact with live elements through the uses of double insulation. These types of equipment are not earthed.
- Class III: These incorporate internal power sources and hence pose less threat to operators.

Further classification is based on the maximal current leakage permissible in the event of malfunction:

- Type B: maybe Class I, II or II. Maximal leakage of 0.5 mA for type I or 0.1 mA for type II.
- Type BF: same as Type B but also incorporates a floating circuit.
- Type CF: this category of equipment is safe to use with direct contact of the heart. A floating circuit is also incorporated, and the maximal permissible leakage current is 0.05 mA for class I and 0.01 for Class II equipment.

Further reading

Anaesthesia UK. Classification of medical equipment. http://www.frca.co.uk/article.aspx?articleid=100734

Answer 25: D

The position of the haemoglobin dissociation curve and thus its tendency to give up and take up oxygen are influenced by many factors.

The curve is shifted to the right (an increased tendency to give up O_2) by any of the following:

- Increase H+
- High CO_2
- High temperature
- Increased 2.3.dpg
- By pregnancy
- At altitude
- Sickle haemoglobin

The curve is shifted to the left (increased affinity for O_2) by any of the following:

- Low PCO_2
- Low H+
- Low temperature

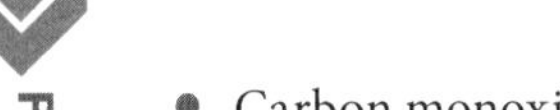

- Carbon monoxide
- Foetal haemoglobin
- Methaemoglobinaemia

Further reading

Power, I., and Kam, P. *Principles of Physiology for the Anaesthetist*. 2nd ed. London: Hodder Arnold, 2008, 135.

Answer 26: C

IV morphine as a bolus would be the best option to treat his acute pain in recovery. Intramuscular (IM) morphine in a distressed child with an IV cannula would be a painful option. Codeine phosphate would be slow to act in this child with severe pain. Post-operative appendectomy patients usually do not require a morphine infusion. The dose of morphine in this child is 100 mcg/kg given as a slow IV bolus.

Further reading

Peck, T.E., Williams, M., and Hill, S.A. *Pharmacology for Anaesthesia and Intensive Care*. Cambridge: Cambridge University Press, 2003.

Answer 27: B

The resulting effect of an electric shock is dependent on the current passing through the victim. High-voltage direct current (DC) causes violent muscle contraction which often results in the victim being thrown from the source. The mains frequency of alternating current (AC) in the United Kingdom (50 Hz) is particularly hazardous but is cheap to produce. An AC of 1 mA produces a tingling, while a current of 3–9 mA is the 'let go' threshold (3 mA in children and up to 9 mA in adults), after which muscle tetany ensues resulting in prolonged exposure. The following list describes consequences at different currents:

- 15 mA: tetany
- 50 mA across the chest: respiratory paralysis
- 100 mA across the chest: ventricular fibrillation

Note that even small currents ('microshocks' of 10–100 μA), if applied directly to the heart via saline drips or pacemaker leads, can induce ventricular fibrillation.

Further reading

Cushing, T.A. Electrical injuries in emergency medicine. *Medscape*. 2010. http://emedicine.medscape.com/article/770179-overview
Yentis, S., Hirsch, N., and Smith, G. *Anaesthesia and Intensive Care A–Z*. 4th ed. London: Churchill Livingstone, 2009.

Answer 28: E

The cranial nerve (CN) pathways involved in brain stem death testing are as follows:

1. Pupillary reflex: afferent CN II and efferent CN III
2. Corneal reflex: afferent CN V and efferent CN VII
3. Vestibule-ocular reflex: afferent CN VIII and efferent CN III
4. Supraorbital pain reflex: afferent CN V and efferent CN VII
5. Gag reflex: afferent CN IX
6. Cough reflex: afferent CN X

Testing also assesses stimulation of respiration by a rising arterial CO_2 tension, by allowing the PCO_2 to rise above 6.65 kP. Hypoxia should be prevented by oxygenation with 100% oxygen prior to the test and by supplying oxygen during the test.

Answer 29: C

The most likely diagnosis of this patient is supraventricular tachycardia (SVT). If this rate does not settle with vagal manoeuvres, then the drug of choice in SVT without severe cardiovascular compromise is adenosine. Adenosine is a short-acting atrioventricular (AV) nodal-blocking agent. Follow-up therapy may consist of diltiazem, verapamil or metoprolol. Amiodarone can be used in SVT that does not involve the AV node. Digoxin would not be the ideal agent in this scenario, nor would DC cardioversion which may be essential in haemodynamically compromised patients. Long-term preventive therapy for such patients would be beta blockers, verapramil and radiofrequency ablation.

Further reading

Peck, T.E., Williams, M., and Hill, S.A. *Pharmacology for Anaesthesia and Intensive Care*. Cambridge: Cambridge University Press, 2003.

Answer 30: B

Awareness during anaesthesia has been reported to occur with an incidence of 0.07% to 0.18%. To reduce this, many methods have been explored with variable outcomes. A clinical method is the PSRT ('pressure, rate, sweating and tears') scoring system which assesses the degree of sympathetic stimulation: P is systolic pressure, R is heart rate, S is sweating and T is tear formation. This system has, however, failed to provide a significant reduction in awareness. Furthermore, concomitant use of drugs such as beta blockers can blunt the sympathetic response in the face of awareness. Several electroencephalographic methods have been developed over the years, including:

1. *Raw EEG (electroencephalogram) analysis*: this employs 19 electrodes and thus is impractical in clinical practice.
2. *Bispectral Index technique*: An EEG is derived using three electrodes attached to the patient's forehead. The signal is analyzed by a complex algorithm to generate a dimensionless value between 0 and 100. The higher the number, the higher the brain activity. Hence, a value approaching 100 corresponds to a fully awake patient and 0 corresponds to no electric activity in the brain. Experimental analysis has indicated that a value between 65 and 85 is consistent with sedation, while a value in the 40–65 range correlates with general anaesthesia. A value below 40 implies burst suppression.
3. *Entropy*: The EEG is chaotic in the awakened patient, and entropy is high. As consciousness decreases, so does the level of disorder. Hence entropy decreases during general anaesthesia.

Further reading

Bruhn, J., Myles, P.S., Sneyd, R., and Struys, M.M.R. Depth of anaesthesia monitoring: what's available, what's validated and what's next? *Br J Anaesth* (2006) 97 (1): 85–94.

PAPER 6 QUESTIONS

Question 1

A 70-year-old man is undergoing a laparotomy for small bowel obstruction. He has a nasopharngeal temperature probe *in situ* that measures 34.8°C. A Baer hugger and fluid warmer are started to correct this hypothermia. Which of the factors below is most responsible for this patient's drop in temperature?

A. Conduction
B. Radiation
C. Evaporation
D. Convection
E. Respiration

Question 2

A 68-year-old man with severe chronic obstructive pulmonary disease (COPD) has been scheduled for a plastic procedure on the ulnar aspect of the hand. Which of the following is the best method for delivering operative anaesthesia?

A. General anaesthesia with muscle relaxant and morphine analgesia
B. Ultrasound-guided interscalene block
C. Ultrasound-guided wrist block targeting the ulnar, medial and radial nerves
D. Ultrasound-guided axillary block targeting radial, ulnar, medial and musculocutaneous nerves
E. Ultrasound-guided targeting of the medial, ulnar and radial nerves at the elbow

Question 3

A 60-year-old woman has had an emergency laparotomy for small bowel obstruction. Her past medical history includes ischaemic heart disease, hypertension and hypercholesterolemia. She had a grade II view of the glottis at induction, and her teeth were in a poor condition. She has had a total of 50 mg rocuronium, with the last dose administered 40 minutes ago. An arterial blood gas (ABG) analysis performed on 40% FiO_2 shows a PaO_2 of 20 kPa and $PaCO_2$ of 5 kPa, with a base excess of –3 mm/L. Which of the following would be an appropriate extubation strategy?

A. Use awake extubation, reverse with neostigmine and use bite block.
B. Use deep extubation to minimize hypertensive response to extubation.
C. Use awake extubation with not more than 80% oxygen to prevent oxygen atelectasis without bite block.
D. Use awake extubation, and avoid reversal agents to prevent tachycardia, hypertension and nausea.
E. Transfer to the intensive therapy unit (ITU) for slow controlled extubation.

Question 4

A 50-year-old man is scheduled for a cystoscopy for recurrent haematuria. He is currently asymptomatic, has no other past medical history and cycles 8 miles daily to and from work. Examination on the morning of his surgery reveals a grade 3 systolic murmur, loudest at the left second intercostal space. How would you proceed?

A. Defer surgery until an echocardiogram (ECG) can be arranged.
B. Defer surgery until a cardiology review is performed.
C. Proceed with surgery with prophylactic teicoplanin.
D. Proceed with surgery with no antibiotic prophylaxis.
E. Proceed with surgery with an arterial line, central venous access, and admit to ITU post-operatively.

Question 5

A 70-year-old man with a history of ischemic heart disease, paroxysmal atrial fibrillation and ventricular tachycardia presents for emergency surgery for a strangulated hernia. You have opted to use the CM5 configuration for intra-operative ECG monitoring because:

A. It allows rapid assessment of arrhythmias.
B. It allows early detection of right coronary perfusion insufficiency.
C. It allows detection of right ventricular perfusion insufficiency.
D. It allows detection of left ventricular perfusion insufficiency.
E. It allows for detection of left ventricular failure.

Question 6

A 69-year-old diabetic patient presents on the emergency list for amputation of a necrotic big toe. His past medical history includes ischemic heart disease, and COPD examination reveals a wheeze throughout the chest and a systolic murmur that is faintly audible. A regional technique is to be used. Which nerves need to be blocked to deliver surgical anaesthesia?

A. Posterior tibial nerve
B. Superficial and deep peroneal nerve
C. Superficial and deep peroneal nerve and posterior tibial nerve
D. Superficial peroneal nerve, sural nerve and posterior tibial nerve
E. Deep peroneal nerve, saphenous nerve and sural nerve

Question 7

A 50-year-old man scheduled for arthroscopy of the knee presents in the pre-assessment clinic. He wants the procedure under a regional technique. His comorbidities include hypertension and mild asthma, and he takes regular bendroflumethiazide 2.5 mg, and salubtamol as needed. Recently he has also started taking aspirin 75 mg once daily. Which of the following pre-operative tests are indicated?

A. Full blood count, urea and electrolytes, clotting screen, ECG and chest X-ray (CXR)
B. Full blood count and urea and electrolytes
C. Clotting screen and CXR
D. Urea and electrolytes and ECG
E. Urea and electrolytes, clotting screen and ECG

Question 8

A 69-year-old man with a history of asthma, diabetes mellitus and hypertension has presented to the emergency department with an episode of syncope. He is complaining of dizziness and shortness of breath, and is unable to remember his date of birth. On examination, he appears pale, with cool peripheries. An ECG shows a bradycardia of 32 beats per minute with type II atrioventricular block. 500 mcg intravenous (IV) atropine was ineffective at improving his rate. Which of the following would be the next most appropriate treatment?

A. Repeat atropine dose to a total of 3 mg.
B. Start an adrenaline infusion at 2 mcg/min.
C. Transcutaneous pacing with sedation and analgesia.
D. Commence an isoprenaline infusion at 5 mcg/min.
E. Transfer to theatre for insertion of a pacemaker.

Question 9

A 29-year-old multiparous woman has had a Caesarean section for foetal distress. Post-delivery, five units of intravenous syntocinon were administered. The surgeon reports ongoing bleeding from the placenta because of reduced tone. Past medical history includes pregnancy induced hypertension for which the patient takes methyl dopa. Which is the next most appropriate strategy to control bleeding?

A. 40 units of syntocinon over four hours
B. A further five units of syntocinon IV
C. Intramuscular (IM) syntometrine (5 mg/500 mcg)
D. IM carboprost
E. A hysterectomy

Question 10

A 66-year-old man is involved in a road traffic accident and has sustained a flail segment rib fracture on the right at the T9–T11 levels. He has no other injuries, and computed tomography (CT) of the head shows no pathology. Which is the most appropriate strategy for analgesia?

A. Avoid non-steroidal anti-inflammatory drugs (NSAIDs) as they impair bone healing.
B. A morphine patient-controlled analgesia (PCA) with paracetamol and an NSAID.
C. A remifentanil PCA with paracetamol and an NSAID.
D. A thoracic epidural with paracetamol and an NSAID.
E. An intercostal nerve block with paracetamol and an NSAID.

Question 11

A 10-year-old child has presented for a tonsillectomy. He is otherwise fit and well. An oral endotracheal tube is to be placed, and thiopentone and atracurium are to be used at induction. What size of a cuffed endotracheal tube and doses of anaesthetic agent would you use?

A. Size 5.5 endotracheal tube, 310 mg thiopentone and 30 mg atracurium
B. Size 6.5 endotracheal tube, 210 thiopentone and 15 mg atracurium
C. Size 5.5 endotracheal tube, 210 mg thiopentone and 5 mg atracurium
D. Size 6.5 endotracheal tube, 210 mg thiopentone and 30 mg atracurium
E. Size 5.5 endotracheal rube, 310 mg thiopentone and 15 mg atracurium

Question 12

A young woman is admitted to the intensive care unit (ICU) after an isolated traumatic head injury. An intracranial pressure (ICP) bolt has been placed, and the neurosurgical team has instructed that the pressure should be maintained below 20 cm H_2O. You have been called to review the patient as the pressure has risen to 30 cm H_2O. Sedation has been instituted with propofol 100 mg/hr which of the following is the next best management option?

A. Increase propofol to 200 mg/hr.
B. Start a remifentanil infusion.
C. Bolus with midazolam.
D. Bolus with thiopentone.
E. Bolus with hypertonic saline.

Question 13

A 30-year-old man, previously fit and well, has been anaesthetized with propofol and fentanyl for an open reduction and fixation of the left tibia. Rocuronium has been used to facilitate tracheal intubation. Diclofenac and prophylactic co-amoxiclav have been given in the anaesthetic room. After transfer to theatre, the blood pressure is 60/30 and he has a tachycardia of 170. Saturation is unrecordable, and he is apnoeic. Ventilation proves very difficult with wheezing throughout the chest. Which agent is most likely to have given rise to these symptoms?

A. Propofol
B. Latex
C. Fentanyl
D. Diclofenac
E. Rocuronium

Question 14

A 67-year-old man is admitted to the intensive therapy unit (ITU) with traumatic brain injury. An ICP bolt is inserted to monitor intracranial pressure. During transfer to computed tomography (CT) imaging, you notice that the ICP rises acutely to 28 mmHg. Which of the following will be your first-line treatment for this?

A. Reduce the positive end-expiratory pressure (PEEP).
B. Ensure the head and neck are in the neutral position.
C. Hyperventilate the patient.
D. Increase FiO_2 to 60%.
E. 100 mL mannitol 20%

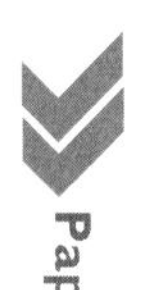
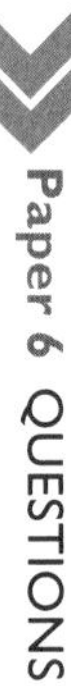

Question 15

There are a wide variety of factors which influence an individual's basal metabolic rate (BMR). In which of the following situations is the BMR likely to be raised the most?

A. Suffering burns over 25% of the body
B. While metabolizing fat
C. Gaining 50% of excess body weight
D. Increasing the body surface-to-weight ratio by 0.5
E. A 10 km race run by a trained athlete

Question 16

A 68-year-old man has undergone a laparotomy for a perforated caecum. Intra-operatively, he was on remifentanil target-controlled infusion. You are considering agents to use for post-operative analgesia. In your knowledge of opioids, which of the following is likely to feature furthest to the right on a dose–response curve?

A. Diamorphine
B. Morphine
C. Fentanyl
D. Remifenanil
E. Pethidine

Question 17

A 50-year-old man who is now in renal failure is intubated and ventilated on the ITU for over a week following initial admission for severe heart failure. His sedation regime consisted of midazolam and morphine. The patient remains apnoeic with a low Glasgow coma score (GCS), despite the infusions being stopped some time ago. Which is the most likely explanation for his prolonged drowsiness?

A. Morphine-6-glucoronide accumulation
B. Hypercapnia
C. Context-sensitive half-life of morphine
D. Intracerebral haemorrhage
E. Accumulation of midazolam metabolites

Question 18

A 24-year-old, 28 weeks pregnant woman attends for a routine antenatal check-up. She has been found to have intra-uterine growth restriction and is advised to give up smoking to improve foetal oxygenation. The foetus receives more oxygenated blood to the head than to the rest of the body. What is the reason for this?

A. Presence of ductus venosus
B. Blood diversion to left atrium via foramen ovale
C. Smoking-induced shift of the haemoglobin dissociation curve
D. Hyperventilation of pregnancy
E. Foetal haemoglobin

Question 19

An 18-year-old male is undergoing an open reduction and internal fixation (ORIF) of a fractured ankle. He had an uneventful anaesthetic for a tonsillectomy at age 6. He has had a rapid sequence induction with propofol and suxamethonim. Opioids were given for analgesia. He is maintained on oxygen, air and isoflurane and paralysed with atracurium. Twenty minutes into the procedure, his end tidal CO_2 ($etCO_2$) begins to rise sharply and his temperature is 39.4°C. He begins to suffer cardiac arrhythmias. ABG analysis shows a metabolic acidosis. Which of the flowing is the most likely cause?

A. Hyperthermia
B. Undiagnosed hyperthyroidism
C. Malignant hyperthermia
D. Underventilation
E. Anaphylactic shock

Question 20

A 60-year-old man is ventilated on the ITU for severe community-acquired pneumonia. An ABG machine calculates the anion gap as 4, 4.2 and 4.3 mmol/l on three occasions. The critical care physician (gold standard) calculates the anion gap as 8 mmol/L. The anion gap value calculated by the blood gas analyser is best described by the following statement:

A. Inaccurate *and* precise
B. Accurate *and* imprecise
C. Accurate *and* precise
D. Inaccurate *and* imprecise
E. Accuracy of 50%

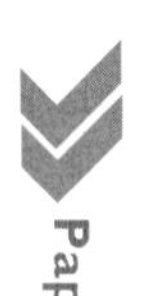

Question 21

An ITU patient is undergoing brain stem death testing. Your consultant opens the eyes and stimulates the cornea of the right eye. The patient blinks, and the result is noted. What are the afferent and efferent limbs of this reflex, respectively?

A. Facial and vagus nerves
B. Facial and oculomotor nerves
C. Trigeminal and oculomotor nerves
D. Trigeminal and facial nerves
E. Trigeminal and oculomotor nerve

Question 22

You are called to review a patient on ITU whose FiO_2 requirement has gradually increased over the last 3–4 hours following the start of nasogastric (NG) feeding at 50 mL/hr. He was spontaneously ventilating on 25% oxygen but now requires a FiO_2 of 55%. You suspect the NG tube is misplaced. Which of the following methods is the most accurate technique for ensuring correct placement of an NG tube?

A. Fast injection of 50 mL of air and listening over the stomach for a gush of air
B. Aspirating fluid and pH testing the aspirate
C. A chest radiograph
D. Injection of saline followed by aspiration of fluid which is pH tested
E. Laryngoscopy to ensure that the NG tube enters the oesophagus

Question 23

A 40-year-old woman is to undergo a laparoscopic left oophorectomy for suspected ovarian cancer. She is very anxious and requests pre-medication prior to anaesthesia on the ward. She is given midazolam pre-operatively and arrives to the anaesthetic room drowsy. During the pre-anaesthetic checks, it is noted that the consent form is missing. It was seen in the notes earlier but now cannot be found. The surgical registrar is happy to document that the consent was taken the night before. What is the best plan of action?

A. Re-consent the patient in the anaesthetic room.
B. Continue with the surgery as the patient was witnessed to have signed the consent.
C. Postpone surgery until tomorrow, and re-consent the patient in the morning.
D. Continue with the surgery, and ask the patient to sign a consent form post-operatively for the records.
E. Ask the patient's husband to sign the consent form.

Question 24

A previously fit and well 35-year-old body builder undergoes endoscopic sinus surgery. He has to be intubated twice as on the first occasion the cuff ruptured. Following extubation, severe laryngospasm ensues. Which of the following techniques to treat laryngospasm is most appropriate at the first instance?

A. Suxamethonium 50 mg IV
B. Propofol 20–50 mg IV
C. Applying continuous positive airway pressure (CPAP) through a facemask with 100% O_2
D. Re-anaesthetizing the patient and inserting a laryngeal mask airway (LMA)
E. Another dose of dexamethasone 8 mg

Question 25

A 27-year-old woman sustains an open fracture to her right ankle. She is otherwise fit and well, and has had previous uneventful general anaesthetics. Anaesthesia is induced, and she is intubated and ventilated. One hour into the start of surgery, you notice the blood pressure is gradually rising. She has a monitored anaesthesia care (MAC) score of 1.5, had 7 mg of morphine 35 minutes ago and had IV paracetamol and diclofenac 45 minutes ago. Her $etCO_2$ has gradually risen from 3.9 to 4.5 kPa over the last half hour. Her temperature is 36.5°C. Which of the following is the most likely cause?

A. Awareness
B. Inadequate analgesia
C. Malignant hyperpyrexia
D. Thyrotoxic crisis
E. Tourniquet pain

Question 26

A 35-year-old woman is undergoing a diagnostic laparoscopy. One hour into the procedure, the surgeons ask for a head-down tilt. Shortly following this, you notice that the patient's saturations drop gradually to stabilize at 92% and that airway pressures increase. Other observations are stable. On examination, there is reduced air entry on the left, and the trachea is central. Which of the following is most likely to be the cause of this?

A. Pneumothorax
B. Migration of the endotracheal tube into the right main bronchus
C. Basal atelectasis
D. Bronchospasm
E. Air embolism

Question 27

A 86-year-old woman with a one-week history of an upper respiratory tract infection is admitted to hospital following a fall. She is found to have a fractured neck of femur. Her oxygen requirements begin to increase gradually over the following 24–48 hours, and she develops confusion and drowsiness. She is intubated and transferred to ITU. On examination, you notice her to have a petechial rash. Her blood tests reveal haemoglobin (Hb) of 11g/dL and platelets of 80 with a white cell count (WCC) of 16. She has a temperature of 36.7°C. Which of the following is most likely to be responsible for her recent clinical findings?

A. Meningitis
B. Thrombocytopaenia purpura
C. Fat embolism
D. Henoch–Schönlein purpura
E. Haemolytic anaemia

Question 28

A young man has undergone prolonged surgery to fix bilateral tibial and ankle fractures. An epidural was sited prior to induction of anaesthesia. Post-operatively, the epidural infusion has been running at 10 mL/hr (0.1% bupivacaine). The patient was comfortable but now has pain in his right calf which is worsening. You are called to review the patient. On examination, the epidural has not migrated and is not leaking, and he has a sensory level to T12 bilaterally with no motor block. Which of the following is most likely to be the cause of his pain?

A. Failure of the epidural
B. Compartment syndrome
C. Inadequate rate of infusion of local anaesthesia
D. Deep venous thrombosis
E. Post-operative oedema

Question 29

A previously well, 28-year-old pregnant woman who is expecting twins and has polyhydramnios is undergoing an emergency Caesarean section under spinal anaesthesia for foetal bradycardia. Immediately following delivery of the second twin, she complains of chest pain, then desaturates, and cardiovascular collapse ensues. She undergoes 6 minutes of cardiopulmonary resuscitation (CPR) following which cardiac output is restored. She develops a petechial rash, and the surgeons report oozing from the tissues. Which of the following is most likely to have occurred?

A. Sepsis
B. Spontaneous pneumothorax
C. Pulmonary thromboembolus
D. Amniotic fluid embolism
E. Acute endocarditis

Question 30

You are called to review a 40-year-old patient on the ward with suspected Guillain–Barré syndrome. The patient reports increasing difficulty breathing, and bedside respiratory function tests show a progressive decline in respiratory function over the last 12 hours. Your consultant decides to admit the patient to the critical care unit. An ABG shows a PaO_2 of 10 kPa and PCO_2 of 7 kPa on 5 L of oxygen. Which of the following is the best mode of ventilation to provide respiratory support?

A. CPAP 5 cm H_2O with FiO_2 50%.
B. Bi-level positive airway pressure (BiPAP) cycling between 12 and 5 cm H_2O with FiO_2 50%.
C. CPAP 10 cm H_2O with FiO_2 50%.
D. Facemask 5l oxygen and repeat an ABG.
E. Intubate and invasively ventilate the patient.

12 PAPER 6 ANSWERS

Answer 1: B

Radiation contributes the most to heat loss during surgeries. At the start of surgery, as the patient is exposed to cold cleaning fluids and cool air flow in the theatre, heat loss exceeds heat production:

- 40% of heat loss occurs due to *radiation* of heat from the body to the environment. The amount and rate of heat loss will depend on the difference between core temperature (body) and the environment.
- 30% of heat loss would occur due to air immediately surrounding the body. The heat loss is proportional to the velocity of air moving around the body. This type of heat loss is called *convection*.
- *Conduction*, in which heat is absorbed by surfaces in contact with the body (e.g. the operating table and fluids), accounts for 5% of heat loss.
- *Evaporation* accounts for 15% of heat loss (e.g. due to cleaning fluids or bowel exposure and from skin).
- Up to 10% of heat loss can occur from the respiratory system due to the cooling effect of anaesthetic gases and vapour.

Answer 2: D

A regional technique would be preferred in this patient. The brachial plexus can be blocked at several sites along its course. The interscalene block is used to provide analgesia for shoulder surgery, distal clavicle and proximal humerus. It often misses the ulnar nerve distribution and hence may have limited use in hand surgery. Furthermore, it can cause an ipsilateral phrenic nerve palsy which would impact respiration. This can sometimes, as in the scenario given here, be undesirable and may lead to further compromise of a failing respiratory system. During hand surgery, surgeons often use a tourniquet which can cause pain. Hence a wrist block or a block at the elbow would be insufficient. The optimal block is an axillary or a supra- or infra-clavicular brachial plexus block. Ultrasound is advocated to reduce the incidence of complications.

Further reading

New York School of Regional Anesthesia. Upper extremity nerve blocks. http://www.nysora.com/files.php?file=Extremity-Nerve-Blocks/NYSORA_UpperExtremityPoster_PRF10aFINAL.pdf

Answer 3: A

The Difficult Airway Society has published guidelines for safer extubation. The process can be classified as low and high risk, based on patient factors (e.g. difficult intubation, anticipated difficult ventilation or airway deterioration). The patient should be prepared for extubation by optimizing temperature and the respiratory, cardiovascular and neuromuscular systems. Attention should also be given to the availability of equipment and assistance. Extubation can then be classified as low or at risk, and the appropriate algorithm followed. This patient is low risk and hence can be extubated. Consideration to transfer a patient to the intensive care unit (ICU) should be given if any systems are suboptimal and can be rectified with time. This patient's gas exchange and cardiovascular system are optimal. The neuromuscular system should also be optimized by reversing the residual neuromuscular blockade, and a bite block should be used. The patient should be oxygenated with 100% oxygen and fully awake prior to extubation to minimize aspiration risk.

Further reading

Difficult Airway Society. Extubation guidelines. 2011. http://www.das.uk.com/guidelines/downloads.html

Answer 4: D

This man has a systolic murmur on the aortic area, which may indicate the presence of aortic stenosis. Other causes for the murmur include an aortic valve sclerosis and a hyperdynamic circulation. This man is asymptomatic and has a good exercise tolerance; hence, it is unlikely that he has significant valvular pathology. Surgery should proceed with meticulous peri-operative care. Haematuria may indicate the presence of a malignancy. He will need an echocardiogram, but this should not delay surgery. Routine antibiotic prophylaxis for endocarditis is no longer advocated. Arterial and central venous catheters are also not required unless he is haemodynamically unstable during the procedure, and he does not need admission to the intensive therapy unit (ITU) if surgery is uneventful.

Further reading

National Institute for Health and Care Excellence. Prophylaxis against infective endocarditis. 2008. NICE guidelines. http://www.nice.org.uk/nicemedia/pdf/CG64PIEQRG.pdf

Telford, R. Valvular heart disease. 2006. http://www.frca.co.uk/article.aspx?articleid=100659

Answer 5: D

In the CM5 lead, configuration is a bipolar lead with the right arm lead placed on the manubrium, the left arm lead placed on the V5 position and the left foot lead placed anywhere else. Lead 1 is selected on the monitor for displaying the electrocardiogram (ECG). It allows for monitoring left ventricular perfusion, and up to 80% of left ventricular ischaemia can be detected. Ischaemia resulting from inadequate perfusion is detected as the ST segment changes. Although arrhythmias can be detected, the primary purpose of the CM5 configuration is to monitor for the development of ischaemic events. Failure of the ventricle cannot be determined from the ECG.

Further reading

Lee, J. ECG monitoring in theatre. *Update Anaesthes* (2000) 11: Article 5, 1–4.

Answer 6: C

The foot is supplied by five nerves. One nerve arises from the femoral nerve, with the other four arising from the sciatic nerve. The sciatic nerve divides into the common peroneal nerve and the tibial nerve variably between the buttock and the popliteal fossa.

Nerves supplying the foot are as follows:

- *Saphenous nerve*: continuation of the femoral nerve, and supplies the lateral aspect of the foot;
- *Deep peroneal nerve*: branch of the common peroneal nerve, and supplies the first web space;
- *Superficial peroneal nerve*: branch of the common peroneal nerve, and supplies the dorsum of the foot;
- *Posterior tibial nerve*: branch of the tibial nerve, and supplies the plantar aspect of the forefoot and sensation to the internal structures of the foot; and
- *Sural nerve*: branch of the tibial nerve, and supplies sensation to the lateral aspect of the foot and the plantar aspect of the hind foot.

Further reading

Loader, J., and McCormick, B. 2008. Anaesthesia for foot and ankle surgery – general and regional techniques. *Update Anaesthes.* http://update.anaesthesiologists.org/wp-content/uploads/2009/10/Anaesthesia-for-Foot-and-Ankle-Surgery.pdf

Answer 7: D

Investigations are often overordered. The National Institute for Health and Care Excellence (NICE) has published guidance on which tests are appropriate based on patient comorbidities and grade of surgery (1–4, with 4 being the most major). This man is undergoing Grade 1 surgery and has asthma and hypertension for which he is taking a diuretic. As such, he would require a urea and electrolytes (U&Es) to monitor for electrolyte imbalance and a baseline ECG. A full blood count (FBC), clotting or chest X-ray (CXR) is not indicated in this circumstance.

Further reading

National Institute for Health and Care Excellence. Preoperative tests: the use of routine preoperative tests for elective surgery. NICE Clinical Guidelines No. 3. 2003. http://www.nice.org.uk/nicemedia/pdf/CG3NICEguideline.pdf

Answer 8: C

This man has a severe bradycardia which has compromised tissue perfusion (syncope, dizziness and cognition). Furthermore, a Mobitz Type II AV block is a risk factor for asystole. Other risk factors include complete heart block, ventricular pauses of greater than 3 seconds and a recent history of asystole. Treatment is insertion of a pacemaker. However, at present he is too unstable for transfer, and interim stabilization measures need to be initiated. Atropine has had little effect, and further doses may not be useful. Although both adrenaline and isoprenaline could be used to improve the heart rate, given the adverse factors in the history, the most appropriate interim measure would be to start transcutaneous pacing in the emergency department. Sedation and analgesia may be required for the patient to tolerate pacing.

Further reading

American Heart Association. American Heart Association guidelines for cardiopulmonary resuscitation and emergency cardiovascular care. Part 7.3: management of symptomatic bradycardia and tachycardia. *Circulation* (2005) 112 (24, Suppl.): IV-67–IV-77.

Resuscitation. Resuscitation guidelines 2012: adult bradycardia algorithm. http://www.resus.org.uk/pages/bradalgo.pdf

Answer 9: D

There are a number of uterotonics available. These include the alkaloid ergometrine which can be administered alone or in combination with oxytocin (syntometrine). It is usually administered as an intramuscular (IM) injection, although it can be given intravenously (IV). It causes an increase in blood pressure, and hence it is not advocated in patients with pre-existing hypertensive diseases. Carboprost, a prostaglandin Fα analogue, does not cause such a hypertensive

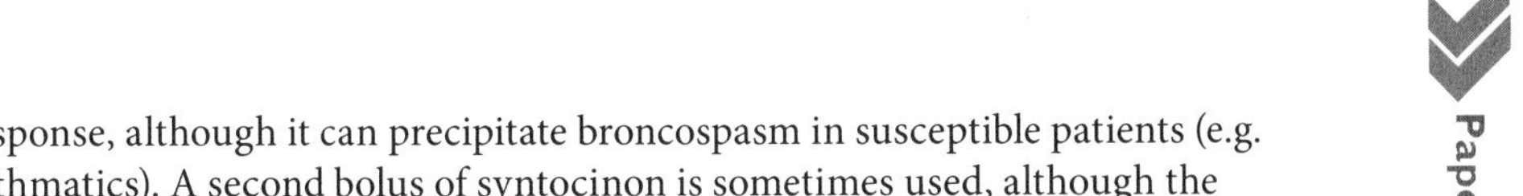

response, although it can precipitate broncospasm in susceptible patients (e.g. asthmatics). A second bolus of syntocinon is sometimes used, although the receptors of the uterus are probably saturated after administration of the first five units. An infusion of syntocinon is used to maintain uterine tone and will not be sufficient in this situation to gain haemostatic control. Misoprostol administered via the rectum can also be used to encourage uterine tone. Surgical techniques such as the B-Lynch suture and hysterectomy are reserved for situations where pharmacological methods have failed.

Further reading

Walfish, M., Nueman, A., and Wlody, D. 2009. Maternal haemorrhage. *Br J Anaesth* (2009) 103 (Suppl. 1): i47–i56.

Answer 10: D

Multiple rib fractures are associated with significant pulmonary comorbidities and mortality, especially in the elderly. Three or more rib fractures in the elderly warrant admission and aggressive analgesia. Consideration should be given to transfer to a trauma centre for management. Pain associated with such fractures induces shallow respiration and suppresses effective cough, thus promoting respiratory tract infection. All patients should have simple analgesics such as paracetamol and non-steroidal anti-inflammatory drugs (NSAIDs), if tolerated. In addition, a patient-controlled analgesia (PCA) system using either morphine or fentanyl should be started for cooperative patients. However, overuse of opioids may further suppress respiratory drive and may increase the incidence of respiratory complications. The best option for the management of severe chest wall injuries is a continuous epidural with local anaesthetic +/– opioid. Although intercostal nerve blocks can be effective, they last only a few hours and will have to be repeated.

Further reading

Trauma.org. Chest trauma: rib fractures & flail chest. http://www.trauma.org/archive/thoracic/CHESTflail.html

Answer 11: B

The initial size of the endotracheal tube selected can be calculated from this formula:

$$(\text{Age} / 4) + 4$$

From this, the correct size of the endotracheal tube is 6.5. However, in clinical practice a 5.5 cuff tube can also be used with the cuff inflated to the correct pressure.

A child's weight is calculated as follows:

- At birth: 3–4 kg
- 1 year: approximately 10 kg
- 0–9 years: age × 2 + 9 kg
- Older than 9 years: age × 3 kg

This gives a weight of 30 kg for a 10-year-old child. (The APLS formula of (age + 4) × 2 kg may also be used.) From this, the following drug calculations may be made:

Thiopentone: 7 mg/kg = 210 mg
Atracurium: 0.5 mg/kg = 15 mg

Further reading

Mitchell, J. 2007. Paediatric anaesthesia. Anaesthesia UK. http://www.frca.co.uk/article.aspx?articleid=100706

Answer 12: C

The aim of treatment is to reduce the cerebral metabolic requirement for oxygen ($CMRO_2$), and to reduce the intracranial pressure. Thiopentone, propofol and midazolam have all been shown to reduce the $CMRO_2$. Opioids have no effect. Increasing the propofol rate will not achieve immediate control, as equilibration will require five half-lives (24 h for propofol). A bolus of propofol can be effective, however. In the options given here, a bolus of midazolam would be the best option. Thiopentone should be reserved for cases refractory to other management strategies, and hypertonic saline is a bridging gap for more definitive surgical therapy.

Further reading

Wijayatilake, D.S., Shepherd, S.J., and Sherren, P.B. Updates in the management of intracranial pressure in traumatic brain injury. *Curr Opin Anaesthesiol* (2012) 25 (5): 540–7.

Answer 13: E

The sudden onset of this clinical presentation suggests anaphylaxis. Neuromuscular blocking agents are responsible for the majority of anaesthesia-related anaphylactic reactions (60%). Most are due to suxamethonium, although in some countries, such as France, rocuronium has been implicated in an equal number of cases.

Further reading

Baillard, C., et al. Case report – anaphylaxis to rocuronium. *Br J Anaesth* (2002) 88: 600–2.

Answer 14: B

When reviewing a patient with raised intracranial pressure (ICP), it is important not to miss the easily correctable causes. The patient should be nursed at a 30° head-up tilt. Ensuring that the head and neck are in the neutral position permits unobstructed cerebral venous return, as does ensuring that the endotracheal tube (if present) is not tied around the neck. Reducing positive end-expiratory pressure (PEEP) also improves venous return. The $PaCO_2$ needs to be kept in the range (4.5–5.0 kPa) as hypercarbia induces cerebral vasodilation. Acute hyperventilation to reduce ICP can be employed to control raised ICP in particular circumstances. However, the risk of inducing hypocarbia-induced cerebral hypoperfusion must be justified. Mannitol and hypertonic saline solutions can also be administered to reduce ICP if the above measures fail.

Further reading

Thavasothy, M. *ICU Notes – Management of Traumatic Head Injury Guidelines as Royal London Hospital*. London: Royal London Hospital, n.d.

Answer 15: E

All of the options given for this question will raise basal metabolic rate (BMR), but by far the greatest increase will be seen in a trained athlete, for trained athletes are said to be able to increase their BMR by as much as 20-fold. Burns are notorious for increasing BMR, but 25% burns is said to increase BMR by 1.18–2.1 times. Increasing the body surface area–to-weight ratio increases radiative heat losses and hence BMR to maintain body temperature. BMR is increased with weight gain.

Further reading

Ganong, W.F. *Review of Medical Physiology*. 22nd ed. New York: McGraw-Hill, 2005, 281–2.

UpToDate. Medline ® abstract for reference 19 of 'Hypermetabolic response to severe burn injury: recognition and treatment'. http://www.uptodate.com/contents/hypermetabolic-response-to-severe-burn-injury-recognition-and-treatment/abstract/19

Answer 16: E

The dose–response curve (DRC) demonstrates the relationship between the dose of a drug (in units) and the desired clinical effect. On a DRC, the further to the right a drug's profile is, the greater the dose of that drug would be to produce the desirable clinical effect (i.e. the less potent it is).

For example, both remifentanil and fentanil are administered in micrograms, but as fentanyl is less potent than remifentanil (a greater dose/kg is needed to produce similar effects), the DRC will plot remifentanil to the left of fentanyl.

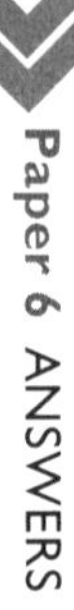

The dose–response curve for the above opioids would follow from left to right – remifentanil, fentanyl, daimorphine, morphine and pethidine. The height of a particular DRC relates to the efficacy, and its gradient indicates the amount of receptors that need to be stimulated before the drug becomes effective.

Further reading

Yentis, S., Hirsch, N., and Smith, G. *Anaesthesia and Intensive Care A–Z*. 4th ed. London: Churchill Livingstone, 2009.

Answer 17: A

The vignette describes the residual effects of the active morphine metabolite morphine-6-glucoronide (M-6-G). M-6-G has a sedative and respiratory depressant effect that can persist for hours after cessation of morphine. M-6-G accumulation is known to occur in renal failure, and hence often the dose of morphine administered is reduced in such patients.

Hypercapnia and CO_2 narcosis can present with drowsiness and apnoeic episodes. However, in ITU such patients would be ventilated until the arterial blood gas (ABG) values qualify the patient for a trial of spontaneous ventilation. The context-sensitive half-life of morphine varies with duration and dose of infusion. However, it is the M-6-G accumulation in renal failure that explains the prolonged drowsiness in the patient discussed here. A cerebrovascular accident can occur but is an unlikely cause here. Midazolam can also accumulate, but it is a less potent respiratory depressant.

Further reading

Travers, A.M. Refresher course: Sedation in the ICU. *S Afr J Anaesthesiol Analg* (2010) 16 (1): 96–100.

Answer 18: B

The most highly oxygenated blood is diverted to the developing brain by the following mechanism. Blood rich in oxygen enters the right atrium and is diverted by the crista terminalis to the left atrium via the foramen ovale. From here, it flows to the left ventricle, out of the aorta and into the carotids, thus ensuring highly oxygenated blood to the brain. The ductus venosus (DV) also shunts oxygenated, but this occurs in the liver where DV shunts oxygenated blood from the placenta into the inferior vena cava, bypassing the liver. Factors affecting haemoglobin and its oxygen-carrying properties will affect foetal oxygenation globally.

Further reading

Yentis, S., Hirsch, N., and Smith, G. *Anaesthesia and Intensive Care A–Z*. 4th ed. London: Churchill Livingstone, 2009.

Answer 19: C

This is a typical presentation of malignant hyperthermia (MH). Underventilation would not explain the pyrexia. Anaphylaxis is possible, but again, such a significant rise in temperature is unlikely. Thyrotoxic crisis should be part of the differential here, but MH should be suspected at the first instance. Hyperthermia (e.g. due to sepsis) may manifest as the scenario given here, but again MH should be your first suspicion.

Further reading

Yentis, S., Hirsch, N., and Smith, G. *Anaesthesia and Intensive Care A–Z.* 4th ed. London: Churchill Livingstone, 2009.

Answer 20: A

Accuracy: refers to how well a value obtained matches the true and actual value
Precision: refers to how closely repeated measurements are similar to each other

In this case, the true value is 8 mmol/L. The measured values, although clustered close to each other (and so precise), are not accurate.

Further reading

Clifton, B., Armstrong S., et al. *Primary FRCA in a Box.* London: Royal Society of Medicine Press Ltd, 2007, 4.

Answer 21: D

This is the corneal reflex. The afferent limb is the trigeminal (ophthalmic division), and the efferent is the facial nerve which supplies the muscles of facial expression.

Further reading

Spoors, C., and Kiff, K. *Training in Anaesthesia: The Essential Curriculum.* Oxford: Oxford University Press, 2010, 541.

Answer 22: C

The gold standard of assessing correct placement of a nasogastric (NG) tube is to perform a chest radiograph, see the NG tube bisecting the carina, leave the oesophagus below the diaphragm and deviate to the left with the tip lying in the stomach. Some hospitals have a policy whereby they are happy to start feeding through an NG tube if the aspirate has a pH compatible with the acidic nature of the stomach (i.e. 5.5 or below). The injection of air as one auscultates over the stomach is a poor indicator of correct NG tube positioning and, according to the National Patient Safety Association, is not safe and must not be used.

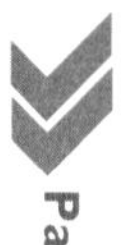

Further reading

Nasogastric tubes 1: insertion technique and confirming position. 2009. http://www.nursingtimes.net/nursing-practice/5000781.article

National Patient Safety Agency. Reducing the harm caused by misplaced nasogastric feeding tubes in adults, children and infants. Patient Safety Alert NPSA/2011/PSA002. 2011. London: NPSA.

Answer 23: C

A sedated patient is not competent to give valid informed consent. The best thing to do in this situation is to postpone surgery until the patient is not under the influence of sedatives and is able to understand, analyse and assimilate information to make an informed decision. The patients' husband cannot consent for the patient unless the patient herself is incompetent and has given power of attorney to her husband. Continuing surgery without a valid consent form is classified as battery under the law unless it is performed in a dire emergency situation as a life-saving measure.

Answer 24: C

Laryngospasm in most cases resolves with the application of simple measures. These should start with suctioning the mouth of any secretions and applying continuous positive airway pressure (CPAP) with 100% oxygen through a facemask held to the patient with a good seal, a firm jaw thrust and the head tilted. If this fails to resolve the issue, a small dose of propofol or suxamethonium may be used (note to keep some anaesthesia on board for the patient if you decide to use suxamethonium). If this is ineffective, it is best to re-anaesthetize and sometimes re-paralyse the patient. The airway can then be maintained with airway adjuncts and supraglottic devices or endotracheal tubes, and extubation can be reattempted immediately or later depending on the cause of the laryngospasm. Dexamethasone can be given to reduce airway oedema, and hence stridor, but only as an adjunct to the other methods to alleviate laryngospasm. The priority is to oxygenate the patient.

Further reading

Spoors, C., and Kiff, K. *Training in Anaesthesia: The Essential Curriculum*. Oxford: Oxford University Press, 2010, 582.

Answer 25: E

This is most likely to be tourniquet pain. Transient hypertension is observed anytime from 30 minutes to an hour into the application of a tourniquet to a limb. It is a diagnosis of exclusion, and requires eliminating the common intra-operative causes of hypertension and tachycardia such as awareness, pain and other less common conditions (e.g. thyrotoxic storm). It is usually resistant to further

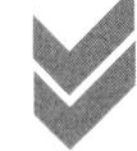

analgesia. This patient is well analgesed and well anaesthetized with a monitored anesthesia care (MAC) score of 1.5. She is otherwise fit and well, so an unexpected thyrotoxic storm is less likely than tourniquet pain. Malignant hyperthermia is a possibility and must feature in your differential, but again is unlikely.

Further reading

Spoors, C., and Kiff, K. *Training in Anaesthesia: The Essential Curriculum.* Oxford: Oxford University Press, 2010, 65.

Answer 26: B

The two most likely causes here are endotracheal tube migration (ETT) migration or a pneumothorax. However, as the trachea is central, ETT migration seems more likely. Basal atelectasis will occur but does not explain the loss of breath sounds over the left lung. Bronchospasm is a possibility; however, there is no wheeze audible, and it is unlikely to be triggered by a change in posture. Air embolism is likely to manifest with a reduction in cardiac output alongside hypoxaemia.

Further reading

Spoors, C., and Kiff, K. *Training in Anaesthesia: The Essential Curriculum.* Oxford: Oxford University Press, 2010, 96.

Answer 27: C

The most likely explanation is fat embolism (FE). It is unlikely that she has developed meningitis, but this should feature in your differential. FE can occur after any traumatic bone injury and is characterized with the escape of fat particles into the systemic circulation where they can act as emboli. The syndrome typically presents 24–72 hours after the insult and is multi-systemic with respiratory (tachypnoea, dyspnoea, crepitations, diffuse lung infiltrates etc.), cardiovascular (tachycardia and ischaemia), central nervous system (CNS) (confusion, headache, coma and retinal infarcts) and skin manifestations (pyrexia and petechial rash). There is no specific test to diagnose FE, but fat particles may be identified in urine, blood, sputum and/or cerebrospinal fluid (CSF). See the reference given here for further detailed information, including Gurd and Wilson's diagnostic criteria. The purpuric syndromes given as possible answers to this question are unlikely to have caused this woman's presentation alone, and a haemolytic anaemia would usually feature a lower haemoglobin (Hb) than 11 g/dL.

Further reading

Spoors, C., and Kiff, K. *Training in Anaesthesia: The Essential Curriculum.* Oxford: Oxford University Press, 2010, 593.

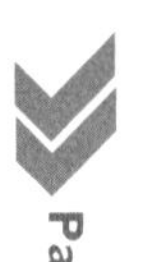

Answer 28: B

Compartment syndrome must be your first differential here. Limb trauma, limb surgery (probably with the use of a tourniquet) and pain not responsive to analgesia should raise strong suspicions. The epidural is unlikely to have failed suddenly, having been running effectively with a sensory block to T12 bilaterally. Epidural and regional anaesthesia do not affect the early diagnosis of compartment syndrome.

Pain in patients with a regional technique can be misinterpreted by the inexperienced as the epidural or regional technique being ineffective rather than the fact that it is effective and the increased pain is a manifestation of compartment syndrome. Hence, vigilance is paramount. The time scale is short for a deep venous thrombosis, although this is not impossible. Post-operative oedema is part of the pathophysiology of compartment syndrome.

Further reading

Spoors, C., and Kiff, K. *Training in Anaesthesia: The Essential Curriculum.* Oxford: Oxford University Press, 2010, 556.

Yentis, S., Hirsch, N., and Smith, G. *Anaesthesia and Intensive Care A–Z.* 4th ed. London: Churchill Livingstone, 2009.

Answer 29: D

This is a typical presentation of amniotic fluid embolism. The risk factors include polyhydramnios, multiple pregnancy and Caesarean section. The pathophysiology is not completely understood. It is thought that during labour or delivery of the baby, foetal fluid, squames and debris cross into maternal systemic circulation, causing cardiorespiratory compromise. However, such fluid, squames and debris are also found in the maternal circulation of those who are asymptomatic. The syndrome presents as an embolic phenomenon, can also trigger an inflammatory response and causes disseminated intravascular coagulation. Sepsis, although a possibility, would cause a more gradual clinical deterioration. A pulmonary embolus is unlikely to explain the petechial rash but should be part of your differential. Acute endocarditis, again, is unlikely to cause a sudden cardiac arrest, having remained asymptomatic antenatally.

Further reading

Moore, L.E. Amniotic fluid embolism. http://emedicine.medscape.com/article/253068-overview

Yentis, S., Hirsch, N., and Smith, G. *Anaesthesia and Intensive Care A–Z.* 4th ed. London: Churchill Livingstone, 2009.

Answer 30: B

This patient has type II respiratory failure. CPAP will improve oxygenation (opening of collapsed alveoli and improvement of functional residual capacity [FRC]) but not significantly improve CO_2 removal. CO_2 removal takes place via an increase in ventilation, which is better provided by bi-level positive airway pressure (BiPAP). BiPAP provides augmentation of the patient's inspiratory effort, allowing a higher tidal volume to be achieved, thus improving minute volume. This patient does not require intubation at this stage, but such an intervention may become necessary if non-invasive measures fail.

Further reading

Anaethesia UK. http://www.frca.co.uk